D1415011

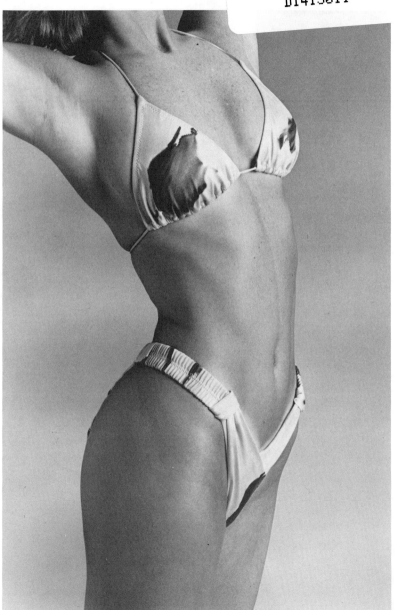

OTHER BOOKS OF INTEREST

BY ELLINGTON DARDEN, PH.D.

The Nautilus Diet

The Six-Week Fat-to-Muscle Makeover

The Nautilus Book (Revised Edition)

The Nautilus Bodybuilding Book (Revised Edition)

New High-Intensity Bodybuilding

100 High-Intensity Ways to Improve your Bodybuilding

The Athlete's Guide to Sports Medicine

Nutrition for Athletes

The Nautilus Nutrition Book

The Nautilus Woman (Revised Edition)

How to Lose Body Fat

32 Days to a 32-Inch Waist

High-Intensity Strength Training

Hot Hips & Fabulous Thighs

For a free catalog of Dr. Darden's fitness books, please send a self-addressed, stamped envelope to Nautilus, P.O. Box 160, Independence, VA 24348.

TWO WEEKS TO A TIGHTER TUMMY

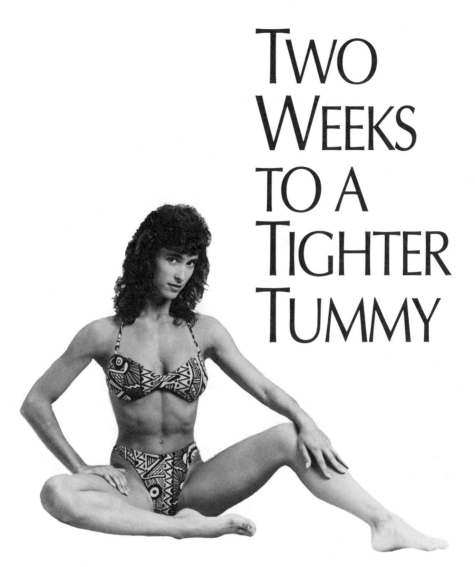

A DAY-BY-DAY 10-STEP PROGRAM

By Ellington Darden, Ph.D.

Taylor Publishing Company
Dallas, Texas

Published by Taylor Publishing Company
          1550 West Mockingbird Lane
          Dallas, Texas 75235

Book design by David Timmons

Library of Congress Cataloging-in-Publication Data
Darden, Ellington, 1943–
     Two weeks to a tighter tummy : a day by day 10 step program / by
Ellington Darden.
          p.   cm.
     ISBN 0-87833-790-3 (pbk.) : $9.95
     1. Reducing diets. 2. Reducing exercises. I. Title.
RM222.2.D296 1992
613.2'5—dc20   91-46775
                                                                 CIP

Printed in the United States of America

10   9

ACKNOWLEDGMENTS

I'd like to thank the following people who helped in the preparation of this book:

Timothy Tew took the exercise and bikini pictures, as well as the front cover of Jill McCann.

Glen Purdy and David Lower took the before-and-after photographs. Glen also planned the food and accessory illustrations.

Tracie Atkinson performed circumference measurements on all the participants.

Karen Coley and Jill Brooks organized and taught the exercise classes.

Terry Duschiniski read the manuscript and offered valuable suggestions.

Jenifer Doherty inputted my handwritten pages into her word processor and made the necessary revisions.

Virginia Brown, R.D., Robert Cade, M.D., Mike Trautschold, and Brenda Hutchins provided dietary help and products.

Lloyd Clarke Sports of Gainesville, Florida supplied Jill McCann's exercise outfit for the cover of the book.

Special appreciation goes to Joe Cirulli and the Gainesville Health & Fitness Center, and to all the women who participated in the research for this project.

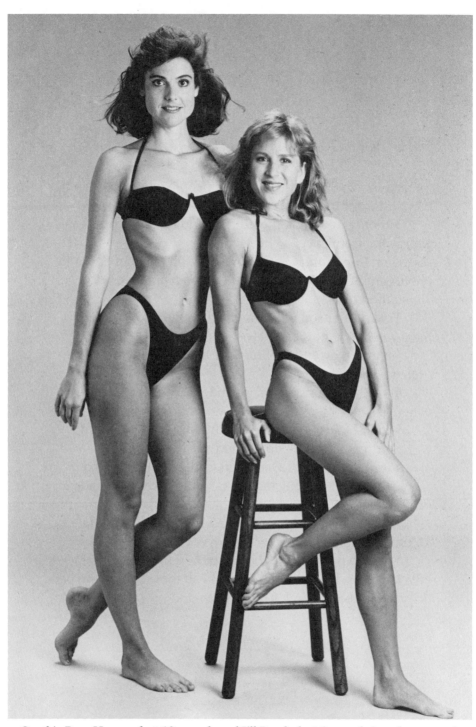

Cynthia Berg-Herman lost 10 pounds and Jill Brooks lost 6 pounds in only two weeks on the Tighter Tummy Program.

CONTENTS

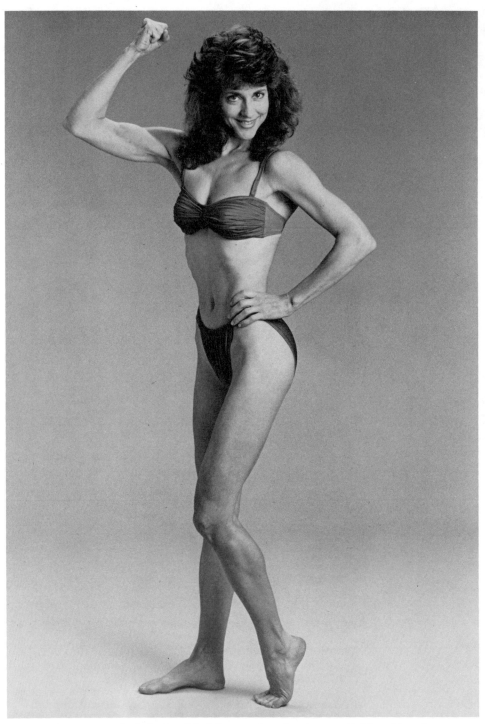

Strong muscles help Cynthia Niemann keep her tummy tight and toned.

CONFUSION ABOUT PROTRUSION

What leads to a tight tummy?

Is it aerobics? Or sit-ups and leg raises? What about a high-fiber diet? Or a low-fat meal replacement? Isn't there a new pill that will melt the flabby fat away? What's the answer?

Most women find that their success rate at getting rid of stomach fat is low at best and counterproductive at worst. Otherwise, there would not be so many diet and exercise gadgets, gimmicks, books, and programs on the market, each new one promising better results than the last.

Certainly, the answer involves dieting and exercising. But which diet and which exercise? Thousands are available.

The diet must be moderately low in calories and well-balanced. The exercise must be intense and progressive.

Even if you spent all your waking hours exercising and only ate small amounts of nature's most nutritious foods, you'd still fall short of your goal. Why?

Because losing fat permanently and firming the underlying tissues require more than diet and exercise. The process necessitates many behavior changes, guided by the best that science has to offer from physiology, sociology, and psychology.

And that's precisely what this book contains. It provides

ten scientific steps to flatten your stomach. Taken separately, each step supplies part of the answer. When they're combined, a synergistic reaction occurs: the total of the steps is greater than the sum of the parts. Synergy is why the program in this book is so result-producing.

SYNERGY AT WORK

I realized I had something very special when I tested the Two Weeks to a Tighter Tummy program at the Gainesville Health & Fitness Center in Gainesville, Florida. Over a period of three months, I supervised 100 women, divided into four groups, through the program.

The first group was composed of twenty-two women. Since I've worked with over 1,500 women in the past on diet and exercise programs, my experience showed that the typical woman in two weeks can expect to lose 4 pounds of fat and 0.83 of an inch off her waist.

Maybe, I thought, with strict supervision, one or two women in the first group would lose more than 5 pounds and more than 1 inch off their waists.

I was elated to find that only one of the twenty-two participants lost less than 5 pounds, and she barely missed the goal by losing 4.76 pounds. Equally impressive was the fact that only two of the twenty-two women lost less than 1 inch from their waists.

BEFORE-AND-AFTER PHOTOGRAPHS

Thumb through the book and you'll notice over a dozen sets of before-and-after photographs that are representative of the women in Gainesville who finished the course. All of the comparison pictures are unretouched. No attempt was made to have the women apply make-up, pose, or smile. They simply had to wear a bikini and stand with their hands on top of their head.

Although each person has unique physical characteristics, each person's body also resembles other bodies in some respect. It will be useful for you to examine these photo-

CYNTHIA NIEMANN

Age: 33

Height: 5'5¹/₄"

Starting body weight: 113.4

Fat lost in pounds: 6

Inches lost from waist: 2

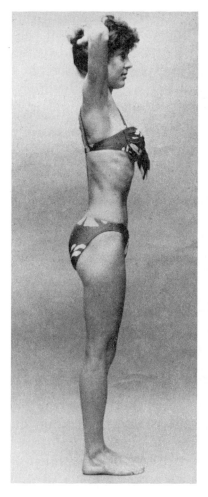 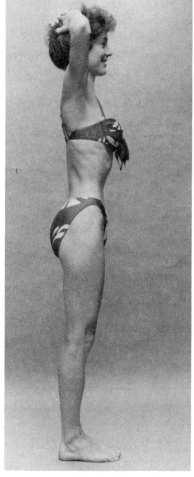

Before　　　　　*After*

graphs carefully with an eye for figure shapes similar to your own. Doing so will help you get a realistic view of what you can achieve.

Notice particularly the waistlines. Some of the women had a small pounds and inches loss, but experienced a large increase in midsection tightness— tightness you can definitely see in the after pictures. This tightness is a result of flabby muscles becoming stronger and better toned. Some of you will see and feel the same thing happening to your waist.

"SO SMALL SO FAST"

Cynthia Niemann was in what many people would consider to be terrific shape. At 5 feet 5¹/₄ inches tall, she weighed 113.4 pounds. At the end of the two-week plan, she reduced her body weight by 6 pounds and lost 2 inches from her tummy. "I never believed my waist could become so small so fast," Cynthia told me. "It's amazing!"

"THE PERFECT TIME IN MY LIFE"

Barbara Worth, married and mother of two teenagers, was another participant in Two Weeks to a Tighter Tummy. After losing 9.47 pounds of fat and 3¹/₂ inches off her waist, Barbara said: "For the last several years my eating and exercising had been poorly planned and badly organized. I needed something to shake me up. That's why this program came along at the perfect time in my life. I'm so thrilled with the results. I plan to continue applying all the steps I learned."

THE PERFECT TIME IN YOUR LIFE

This program can also happen at the perfect time in your life. Do ordinary diets have little effect on your tummy fat? Is middle protrusion your figure flaw? Do you wish you could wear body-revealing fashions instead of belly camouflage? Or do you just want to lose a few pounds quickly?

If you answered *yes* to any of these questions, this book is for you.

Read and apply it, NOW!

BARBARA WORTH

Age: 47

Height: 5'7"

Starting body weight: 138.5

Fat lost in pounds: 9.47

Inches lost from waist: 3$\frac{1}{2}$

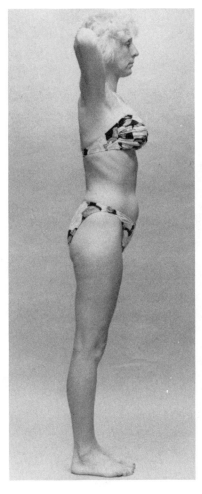

Before

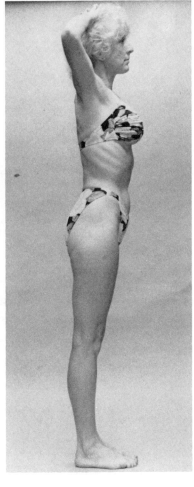

After

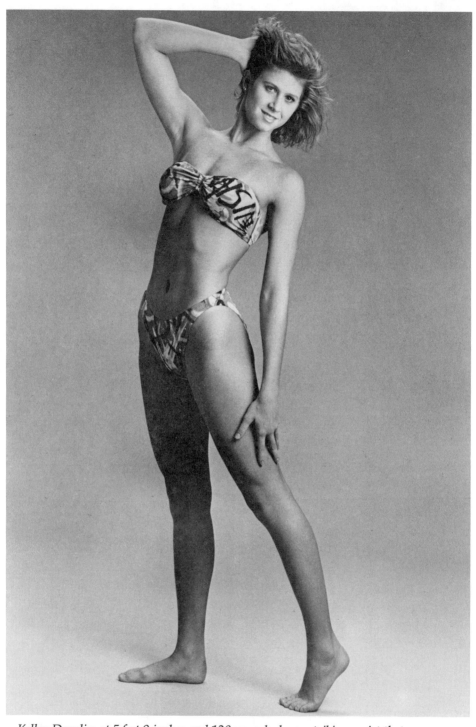

Kelley Donelin, at 5 feet 9 inches and 128 pounds, has a striking waist that measures 24 inches.

WHAT TO
EXPECT

Whati can you expect if you follow the Tighter Tummy Program exactly as directed for 14 days? An examination of the average losses of the women that I supervised through the plan should provide the answer.

AVERAGE EXPECTATIONS

During the spring of 1991, the two-week program was tested with one hundred women from the Gainesville Health & Fitness Center in Gainesville, Florida. Statistics show that the average woman was 33.44 years old, 64.78 inches tall, and had a starting body weight of 134.76 pounds.

Each woman involved in the research lost an average of:

- 7.02 pounds of fat
- 1.83 inches off the waist
- 0.80 inches off the hips
- 1.37 inches off the thighs

The women simultaneously built an average of 1.26 pounds of muscle, which not only made them look better, but raised their metabolic rates by almost 100 calories per day. The above losses and gains are average expectations for a typical woman who follows the program.

MARY SMITH

Age: 33

Height: 5'4½"

Starting body weight: 122.5

Fat lost in pounds: 8.01

Inches lost from waist: 2

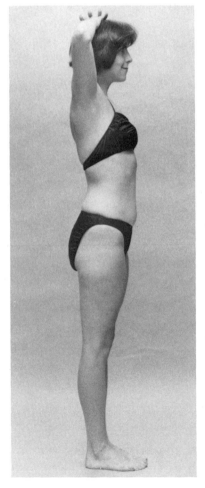 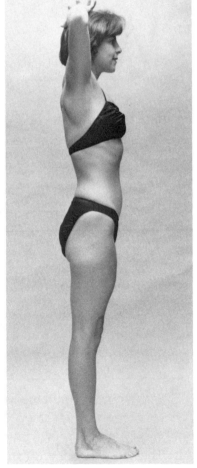

Before   *After*

HIGHER EXPECTATIONS

On the other hand, many women exceeded the average. The most pounds and inches lost by any of the 100 women were as follows:

- 10.36 pounds of fat
- 3.5 inches off the waist
- 3.25 inches off the hips
- 3.25 inches off the thighs

SERIOUS GOALS

If you're a thirtysomething woman who is about 5 feet 5 inches tall and weighs approximately 135 pounds, you can expect to lose 7 pounds of fat and almost 2 inches off your waist. As a result, you'll most definitely have a tighter tummy.

If you weigh significantly more or less than 135 pounds, your overall results may vary considerably. The principles involved in this book still apply. You may be one of the women who gets greater-than-average results.

The older you are, however, the tougher it is to flatten your midriff. At forty-five years and older, a woman can achieve some fairly dramatic results. But she may have to accept a less than board-flat belly, especially if she's had a few pregnancies.

On the other hand, many younger women become obsessed with their bodies. You've probably met some of them, those who diet and exercise all the time to be *thin* and *perfect*. Their entire self-image is wrapped up in their looks. Sure, caring about your body is healthy and positive. Just don't take the concern to an extreme.

REALISTIC ACTION

Be realistic. That's what this course is about—*reaching realistic goals.*

If you follow the course of action throughout this book, you'll have a waistline you can be proud of and a figure to match.

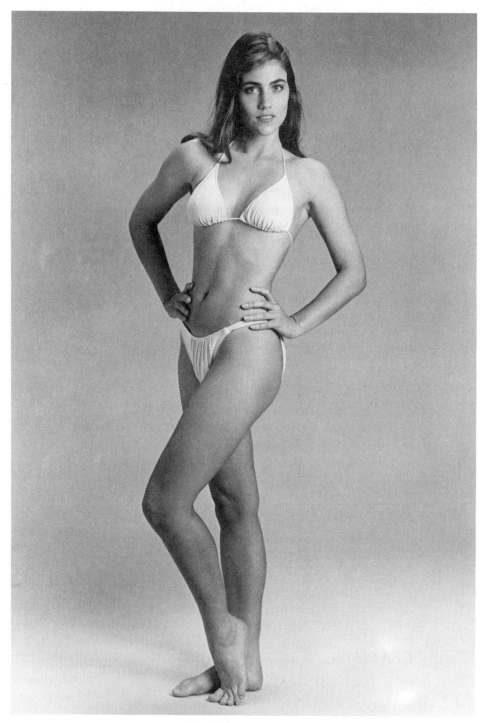

Kelli Jones went through the two-week plan and built 2¹/₂ pounds of bodyshaping muscle.

THE TEN-STEP PROGRAM

Y ou probably don't need a technical explanation of the muscles ir lved and their relation to the internal organs to realize wha. ɔu're doing to yourself by walking around with a fat stomach. You're already unhappy about your shape and aren't interested in whether the protrusion has overstretched the *rectus abdominis*, the *external oblique*, or the *transverse abdominis*.

You just want to make your tummy smaller and tighter. You want to be able to pull it in and make it flat.

Two Weeks to a Tighter Tummy does just that. It supplies all the ingredients to tighten your tummy and make it smaller—quickly.

Almost every day for two weeks, you'll be instructed through ten steps—ten steps that zero in on the gut of the matter. Before I get into full chapter explanations of each step, a preview will prepare you for what's ahead.

STEPS TO A TIGHTER TUMMY

Step 1 and Step 2 present a tried-and-proven, low-calorie, carbohydrate-rich diet divided into four or five small meals a day. You'll experience virtually no hunger on such an eating schedule as you watch the pounds and inches disappear from your waist.

Step 3 regulates your intake of salt. Salt is 40 percent sodium and 60 percent chloride. The sodium in salt is the main concern when it comes to high blood pressure and excessive fluid retention, which concern many women. Salt also stimulates your appetite. Most women consume several times as much salt (sodium) as they need each day. Step 3, therefore, keeps your sodium intake at 2,400 milligrams or less per day.

Step 4 promotes drinking from one to one-and-one-quarter gallons of water a day. Large amounts of this natural fluid accelerate the fat-loss and tummy-tightening process. A little-known scientific fact reveals that the body requires 227 calories to warm one gallon of ice water to core body temperature. You'll discover how to use this fact to your benefit.

Exercise, to be most effective, should be performed with the least amount of momentum involved in the movement. The best way to do this is by lifting and lowering your body weight slowly. This is described and illustrated in Steps 5 and 6. You'll be amazed at the muscle isolation and body-part tightening possible from a few simple exercises. Best of all, you'll feel and see the results from the very first workout.

Step 7 shares with you a technique called the stomach vacuum, which has been used for years by professional bodybuilders to tighten and define their midsections. You're only a few deep breaths away from learning and applying this trade secret.

What could be simpler than taking a brief walk after your evening meal? Research proves that doing so can speed up the burning of belly fat, as you'll experience in Step 8.

Step 9 stresses the importance of rest and sleep. A proper balance between work and recovery is necessary for maximum fat-loss results.

Step 10 addresses various fat-loss problems with scientific facts. For example, you'll understand why it's to your advantage to sleep cool. You'll also learn why and how to use particular colors of tablecloths and plates to appease your appetite.

ANGIE THOMAS

Age: 36

Height: 5'5"

Starting body weight: 124.7

Fat lost in pounds: 5.9

Inches lost from waist: 2⁵/₈

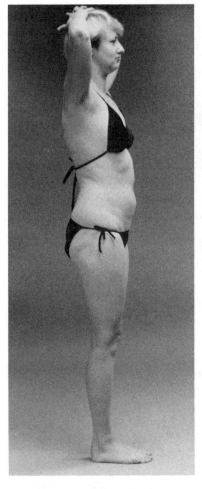 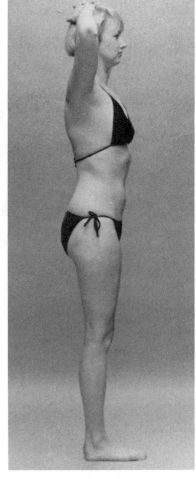

Before   *After*

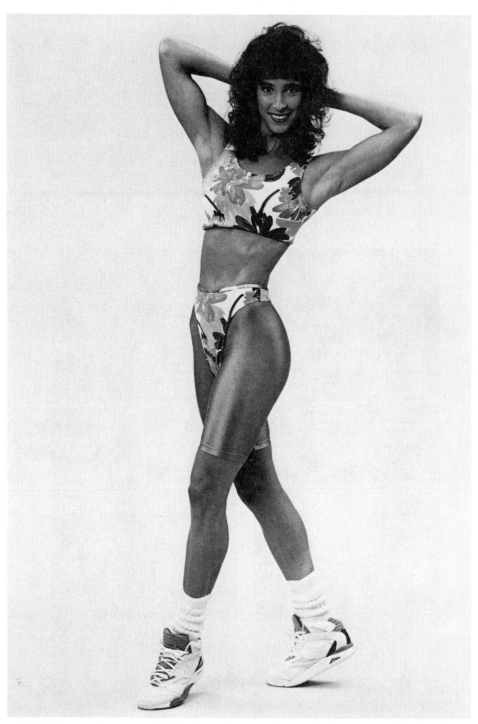

Jill McCann, whose superfit body is on the cover, knows the importance of keeping her muscles strong.

ONLY TWO WEEKS

Through these ten steps you'll be directed in how to use the recommended foods, meals, recipes, exercises, and actions that do the most dramatic job on your stomach as easily, efficiently, and quickly as possible. Of course, in the process, the rest of your body will be strengthened and re-shaped too.

In only two weeks you can make significant changes in the way your tummy looks, feels, and functions.

Say *yes*, now!

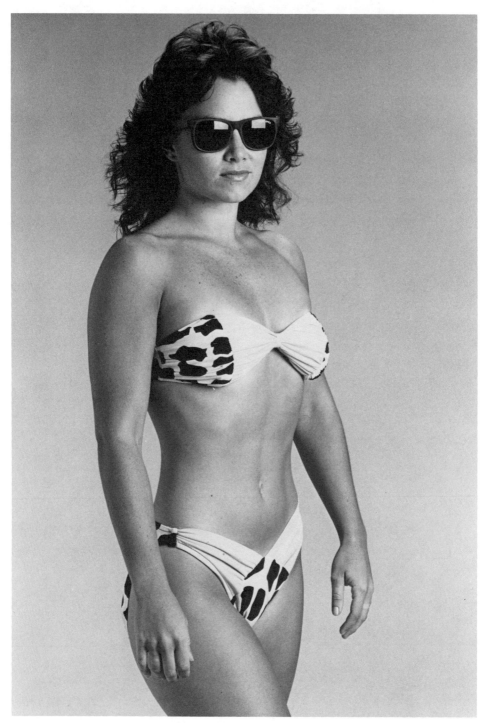

Stephanie Freas reshaped her body for the beach by losing 7.77 pounds of fat.

BEFORE GETTING STARTED

B efore starting to make your tummy tighter and smaller, there are a few things that you need to do.

CONSULT WITH YOUR PHYSICIAN

Be sure your doctor knows you are going on this ten-step program for 14 days. Let him examine this book so he understands what's involved. He may want to give you a physical if he hasn't given you one in the last year.

There are a few people who should not try the program: children and teenagers; women with certain types of heart, liver, or kidney disease; diabetics; and those suffering from some types of arthritis. The diet is also too low in calories for most men. This should not be taken as an all-inclusive list. Some women should follow the course only with their physician's specific guidance and recommendations. Consult your doctor beforehand to play it safe.

FIND A FRIEND TO GO THROUGH THE PROGRAM WITH YOU

Although it is certainly possible to get great results going through the course by yourself, you'll probably lose more inches and pounds if you team up with a friend or several friends. You and your friend should try to shop together, exercise together, walk together, and share each other's problems.

DO BODY PART MEASUREMENTS

You and your diet partner can best do the measurements together. In a private room, slip on your smallest bikini. A bikini works better than a one-piece bathing suit because it reveals your entire midsection. With a bathroom scale and a plastic tape measure, record the following relaxed measurements:

	Before	*After*	*Difference*
Body weight	_____	_____	_____
High waist (two inches above navel)	_____	_____	_____
Waist (at navel level)	_____	_____	_____
Low waist (two inches below navel)	_____	_____	_____
Hips (at largest protrusion with heels together)	_____	_____	_____
Right thigh (just below buttocks crease)	_____	_____	_____
Left thigh (just below buttocks crease)	_____	_____	_____

JILL BROOKS

Age: 25

Height: 5'4"

Starting body weight: 120.9

Fat lost in pounds: 6.69

Inches lost from waist: 1$\frac{1}{2}$

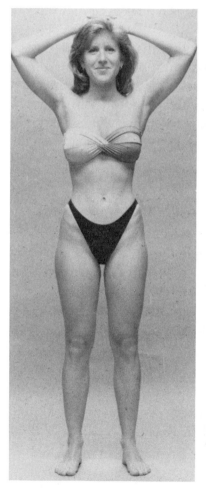

Before

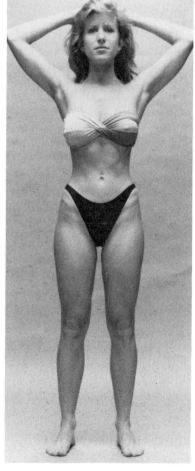

After

Take all your measurements standing with your weight equally distributed on both feet. Apply the tape firmly, do not compress the skin, keep it parallel to the floor, and record the measurement to the nearest $1/8$ inch.

In my previous diet and exercise books, which involve six- and ten-week programs, I always recommend the use of an at-home pinch test to determine body fat percentage. However, a pinch test using your thumb, first finger, and a ruler is not sensitive enough to determine significant differences over just two weeks. Metal skinfold calipers, which are often found at fitness centers, may be used if available. Otherwise, an at-home pinch test is not necessary for this program.

Although two weeks is a short time, before-and-after pictures of yourself in a bikini can still prove meaningful. Stand against an uncluttered background with your hands on your head and feet apart evenly. Do not suck in your stomach. A front and a side pose taken two weeks apart will provide interesting comparisons, especially if you lose significant pounds and inches.

CHECK OUT YOUR FAVORITE SUPERMARKET

The two-week eating plan in this book is the simplest diet that I've ever designed. It also requires the least amount of preparation. Furthermore, all of the foods can be purchased from almost any large supermarket. You will need, however, to become well-acquainted with certain sections of the store.

For breakfast, you'll have a choice of some of the following foods:

- Vanilla Go!, a quick-shake-in-a-carton manufactured by Phoenix Advanced Technology
- DynaTrim Instant Meal, a powder that mixes with skim milk
- Reduced-calorie bread

- Heart Beat, a corn-oil spread manufactured by Nucoa

For lunch, make sure the following foods are available:

- Light Balance, Chicken Fiesta with Beans and Rice, a Lunch Bucket microwave meal manufactured by Doubletree Foods
- Healthy Choice, Spicy Chili with Beans and Ground Turkey, a microwave meal manufactured by Conagra
- Refrigerated white meat, chicken or turkey, 10 calories per slice

For dinner, you'll have a choice of certain Healthy Choice frozen dinners and Healthy Choice frozen entrees. Both are usually located in separate sections of the frozen food aisle.

Other foods— such as fruits, yogurt, skim milk, and soft drinks— should be easy to find. Read through the complete eating plan before you visit the supermarket.

TAKE A VITAMIN-MINERAL TABLET EACH DAY

You should take *one* multiple vitamin-with-minerals tablet each morning of this two-week eating plan. The tablet should contain calcium and iron. Study the label, however, and make sure no nutrient exceeds 100 percent of the U.S. Recommended Daily allowances. High-potency supplements and super-stress formulas are a waste of money.

AVOID STRENUOUS ACTIVITY ON YOUR OFF DAYS

The primary exercise program in this book consists of workouts on three non-consecutive days each week. On the off days it is important to rest and relax. No other strenuous exercise or activity is permitted.

Research shows that too much exercise can be more harmful to your system than too little exercise, especially

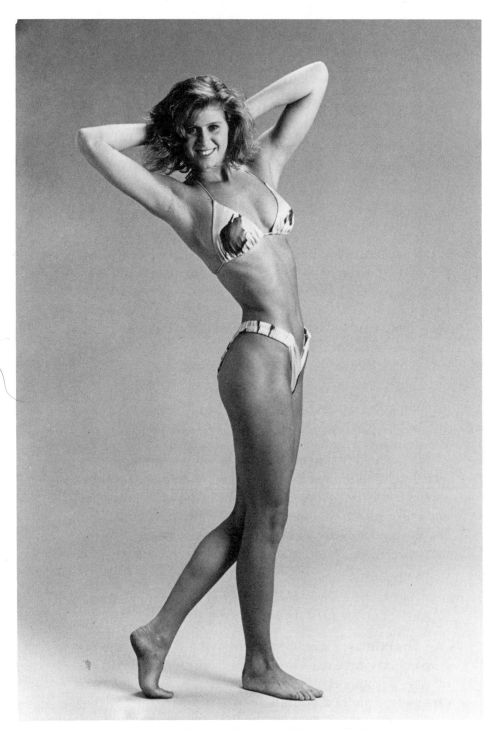

Tall, lean Kelly Donelin is an avid basketball player.

when you are following a low-calorie diet. Rather than lose fat, your body can actually start preserving it.

Two women who were a part of the last group of research participants at the Gainesville Health & Fitness Center didn't believe me when I warned them about the problems of over exercising. Both continued to exercise vigorously on their off days. To their surprise, but not mine, neither managed to lose any fat over the 14-day program.

Don't let yourself fall into this category. Follow the plan exactly the way it is described to maximize your fat loss.

GET SERIOUS

You've familiarized yourself with what to expect and taken all the precautionary measures, now it's time to get serious. It's time to slim down and tighten up by applying Steps 1 through 10.

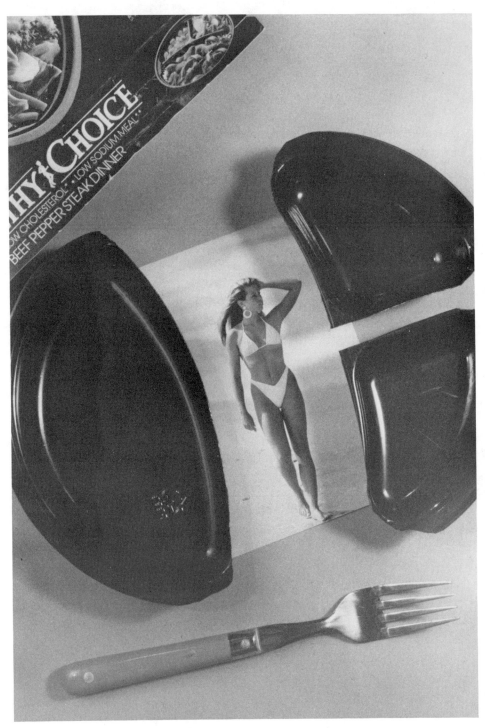

Frozen microwave meals—less than 400 calories each—are an essential feature of the Tighter Tummy Eating Plan.

STEP 1

Eat Smaller Meals More Frequently

If your goal was to get as fat as possible, in the most efficient manner, you'd be wise to eat one very large meal each day immediately before going to bed. In other words, you'd eat for only one hour out of every twenty-four. And that one hour would always precede sleep.

Sounds ridiculous, doesn't it? Who in their right mind would want to get as fat as possible?

FAT-FORMING EATING HABITS

In actuality, many Americans have eating patterns that are not all that different from the above example. It's a pattern of: no time for breakfast, work through the lunch hour, eat a big dinner, and snack nonstop until bedtime. Millions of Americans starve their bodies when they most need calories and stuff them when they'll be doing nothing more strenuous than reading the newspaper and watching TV. Such eating habits make no sense, unless you're trying to weigh as much as possible.

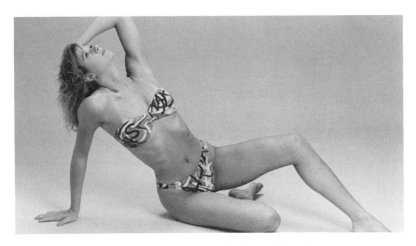

Strong lean bodies look terrific from all angles

SMALL MEALS MAKE SENSE

Research shows that losing fat in the most efficient manner requires just the opposite—eating smaller meals more frequently. Large meals stimulate excessive insulin production and insulin is your body's most powerful pro-fat hormone. Small meals bring on small insulin responses. Thus, it is advantageous to consume many smaller-than-average-sized meals per day.

It makes little difference, however, whether you consume four, five, or six small meals a day, as long as you are eating every three to five hours that you are awake. It is also necessary to limit any meal to 500 calories or less.

The meal pattern for the Tighter Tummy Diet is illustrated below.

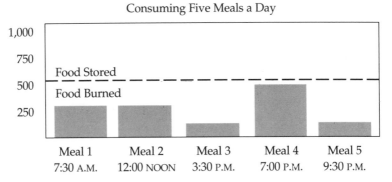

Consuming Five Meals a Day

The Tighter Tummy meal pattern involves a 250-calorie breakfast, a 250-calorie lunch, a 100-calorie afternoon snack, a 400-calorie dinner, and a 100-calorie late-night snack. Women who weigh over 120 pounds should consume all five meals each day for fourteen days. Women under 120 pounds should omit the late-night snack.

FOUR OR FIVE

Remember, four or five small meals a day—with none of the meals exceeding 400 calories—is the best way to lose fat.

Keep your meals small and your fat loss will be large.

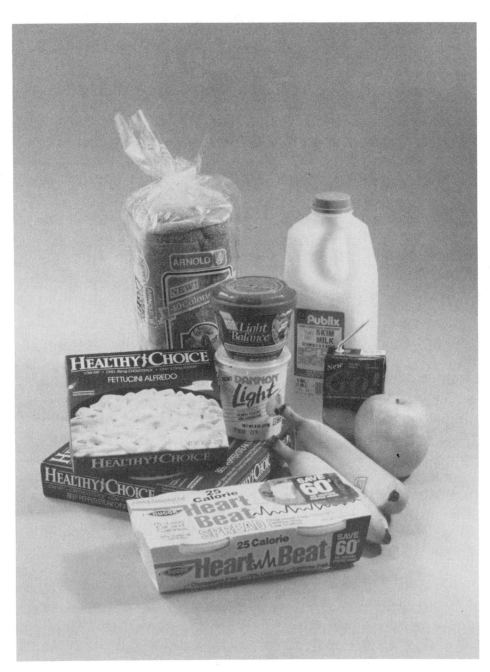

A selection of foods from Step 2.

Lunch, 250 calories.
Select one of the four following meals with listed foods:

1. Light Balance (Lunch Bucket) Chicken Fiesta
    Microwave Meal (210)
    1 slice reduced-calorie bread (40)
    Noncaloric beverage

2. Healthy Choice Spicy Chili with Beans and
    Ground Turkey Microwave Meal (210)
    1 slice reduced-calorie bread (40)
    Noncaloric beverage

3. Sandwich
    2 slices reduced-calorie bread (80)
    2 teaspoons Heart Beat spread (17)
    2 ounces white meat (about 8 thin slices),
    chicken or turkey (80)
    2 slices tomato (14)
    2 lettuce leaves (4)
    $^1/_2$ medium (8 $^3/_4$-inch) banana (50)
    Noncaloric beverage

4. Chef Salad
    1 cup lettuce, chopped (10)
    2 slices tomato, chopped (14)
    1 ounce cheese (regular, not diet) (100)
    2 ounces white meat, chicken or turkey (80)
    1 tablespoon diet dressing (6)
    1 slice reduced-calorie bread (40)
    Noncaloric beverage

Mid-afternoon Snack, 100 calories.
Select one:

1 medium (8 $^3/_4$-inch) banana
1 apple (3-inch diameter)
$^1/_4$ cup (2 small boxes) raisins
8 ounces light, nonfat, flavored yogurt

Dinner, 400 calories.

Select one of the seven following Healthy Choice Frozen Dinners or Entrées with the listed foods:

1. Beef Pepper Steak Dinner (290)
    2 teaspoons Heart Beat spread (17)
    1 cup skim milk (90)
    Noncaloric beverage

2. Salisbury Steak Dinner (300)
    1 teaspoon Heart Beat spread (8)
    1 cup skim milk (90)
    Noncaloric beverage

3. Chicken Enchilada Dinner (330)
    1 teaspoon Heart Beat spread (8)
    $^2/_3$ cup skim milk (60)
    Noncaloric beverage

4. Breast of Turkey Dinner (290)
    2 teaspoons Heart Beat spread (8)
    $^2/_3$ cup skim milk (60)
    Noncaloric beverage

5. Shrimp Creole Dinner (230)
    2 slices reduced-calorie bread (80)
    3 teaspoons Heart Beat spread (25)
    $^2/_3$ cup skim milk (60)
    Noncaloric beverage

6. Lasagna with Meat Sauce (in entrée section) (250)
    1 slice reduced-calorie bread (40)
    2 teaspoons Heart Beat spread (17)
    1 cup skim milk (90)
    Noncaloric beverage

7. Fettucini Alfredo (in entrée section) (240)
    2 slices reduced-calorie bread (80)
    2 teaspoons Heart Beat spread (17)
    $^2/_3$ cup skim milk (60)
    Noncaloric beverage

Evening Snack, 100 calories.
Only for women weighing over 120 pounds. Select one:

> 1 medium (8 $^3/_4$-inch) banana
> 1 apple (3-inch diameter)
> $^1/_4$ cup (2 small boxes) raisins
> 8 ounces light, nonfat, flavored yogurt

IMPORTANT NOTES FOR THE TIGHTER TUMMY DIET

- The Vanilla Go! Quick-Shakes are sold in a shelf-stable, rectangular, three-pack. Each serving contains 8 fluid ounces and comes with a plastic straw. Simply refrigerate and consume directly from the carton. Or you may pour Go into a blender with several ice cubes and a packet of Equal and mix for a thicker drink. Go also is sold in chocolate flavor, but the calories are significantly higher.

- The DynaTrim Instant Meal is a powder that mixes well with skim milk. It tastes better cold, and ice cubes may be blended with it also. Several flavors are available and they may be used as long as the calories per serving (without skim milk) are 100. Read the labels carefully!

- If Go and DynaTrim are *not* available in your supermarket, you may substitute Carnation Instant Breakfast or Ultra Slim-Fast. Just make certain the powder plus the skim milk contains 190 calories. Once again, read the product labels carefully.

- There are many reduced-calorie breads, at 40 calories per slice, that are sold in your supermarket. Try to select one that is high in fiber.

- Heart Beat spread has a great taste, but because of its high water content, it doesn't melt like regular butter or margarine. However, it still spreads on bread or toast. Do not cook with it or try to use it in a microwave oven. If bread is not called for in the dinner you choose, mix the Heart Beat into the vegetables.

- Noncaloric beverages are any type of water—tap, bottled, mineral, carbonated, or flavored—with no calories. With bottled water, make sure the sodium and salt content are very low. Other noncaloric beverages are soft drinks with zero or only 1 calorie per serving, and decaffeinated teas and coffees. Try to avoid regular coffee and tea with caffeine for two weeks, if possible. Caffeine is a strong stimulant, as well as a diuretic.

- The Light Balance (Lunch Bucket) Chicken Fiesta Microwave Meal is sold in a shelf-stable, 8.25 ounce, blue container. The Healthy Choice Spicy Chili with Beans and Ground Turkey Microwave Meal is similar, except it's in a green package. Both heat quickly in a microwave oven and are very tasty and filling.

- One of the lunch choices, the white meat sandwich, includes a 50-calorie fruit: $1/2$ medium ($8^3/4$-inch) banana. You can keep the other half of the banana fresh by wrapping it tightly in aluminum foil and freezing it. Be sure and peel the banana before you freeze it or the peeling will turn an undesirable color. A banana is a great taste-treat when frozen.

- The Healthy Choice dinners and entrées that are used for your evening meals are all nutritious and delicious. The women on the Tighter Tummy Program in Gainesville loved them. To heat, you may use a microwave or conventional oven. Follow the directions on the container. And don't forget to add the other foods, especially the Heart Beat spread, to the Healthy Choice selections. The Heart Beat spread adds satiety value to the meal in the form of fatty acids. Do not omit it.

- Try all the Healthy Choice recommendations over the first week before you select only your favorites. Variety is important in dieting.

- Calories are important, too. Make sure you correctly use measuring spoons, cups, and food scales in your meal preparation. And don't forget to read all your food labels thoroughly.

- Remember, this is a two-week, 1,000-calorie-a-day diet for women who weigh under 120 pounds. For women above 120 pounds, the diet is 1,100 calories per day. The only difference between the two diets is the added 100-calorie evening snack for women over 120 pounds.

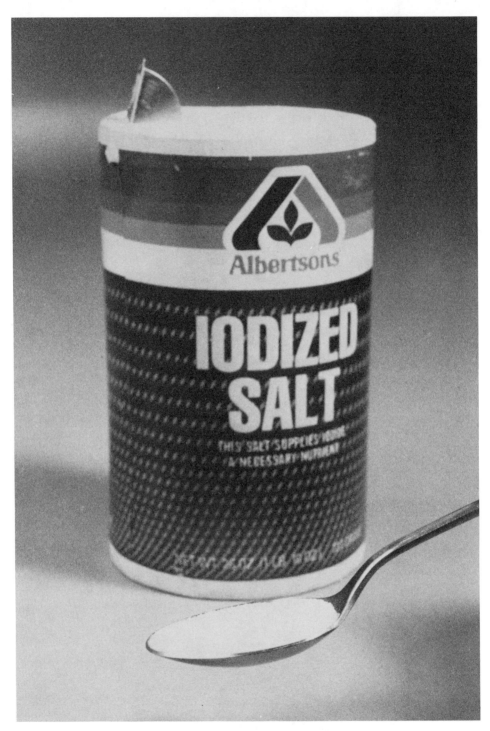

Your salt intake will be limited to approximately one teaspoon per day.

STEP 3

Reduce Your Salt (Sodium) Intake

Here's a quick quiz. Rank the following foods from most salt to least salt:

❑ 6 ounces of V-8 juice
❑ $^1/_2$ cup Jell-O Instant Chocolate Pudding
❑ 1 cup of Total cereal
❑ 1 small bag of potato chips
❑ 1 ounce of salted peanuts

Here are the answers in milligrams of sodium: V-8 = 555, pudding = 460, cereal = 375, chips = 133, and peanuts = 123. The listings from top to bottom are the correct rankings. The V-8 juice has over twice as much sodium as the chips and nuts combined. Taste and visible salt are not always reliable indicators.

SODIUM FACTS

The Food and Nutrition Board's National Research Council recommends 1,100 to 3,300 milligrams of sodium daily for adults. These levels are equivalent to $^1/_2$ to $1\,^1/_2$ teaspoons of table salt. However, the average American consumes many times more sodium than required each day.

TERESA LISCHKA

Age: 30

Height: 5'0¼"

Starting body weight: 112.1

Fat lost in pounds: 6.3

Inches lost from waist: 2⅝

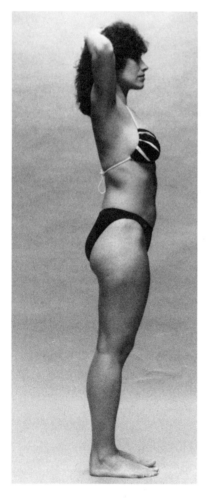

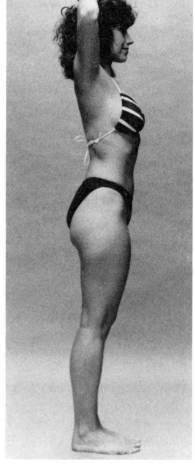

Before *After*

What's the problem with getting too much salt and sodium in your diet? Aside from the relationships between excessive sodium and high blood pressure, excessive sodium and fluid retention, salt generally hangs out with high-calorie foods. There seems to be an almost irresistible urge to eat foods that contain salt, fat, and sugar. And once you start, it's difficult to stop.

SAY GOODBYE TO THE SALT SHAKER

Hide your salt shaker. You won't need it for the next two weeks.

Even though most processed and frozen foods are high in sodium, this is not the case with the Tighter Tummy Diet. One factor in selecting the foods on this eating plan is their low-sodium content.

On the Tighter Tummy Diet, none of your daily menus contains more than 2,400 milligrams of sodium, and this is plenty of sodium for even the most active woman.

Furthermore, your waistline will notice the difference almost immediately.

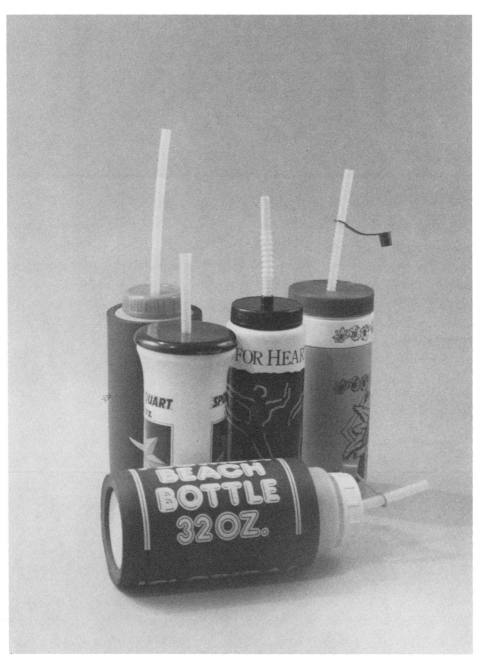

For the next two weeks, a water bottle will be one of your best friends.

STEP 4

*Drink One to One-and One-Quarter
Gallons of Water per Day*

At a glance, you can tell the women who have
been through the two-week program in Gainesville, Florida.

Yes, they are the ones with the small, tight tummies. But
they are also the ones sipping water all day from a 32-ounce
insulated container with a plastic straw poked through the
lid.

A MAGIC POTION?

Water will do more to generate fat loss than any other
single, simple thing you can do. There is no such thing as a
magic fat-loss potion, but water comes pretty close.

Your cells are like plants that thrive in a rain forest—
they crave water. Only when they are fully hydrated does
your body function optimally.

If you don't drink enough water, your body's reaction is
to retain the water it does have. This, in turn, hampers kidney
function and waste products accumulate. Your liver is then
called on to flush out impurities. As a result, one of your liver's main functions—metabolizing stored fat into usable energy—is minimized.

Water can be used to drown food cravings, too. It gives you a sense of fullness, and as a result, you consume fewer calories.

STANDARD RECOMMENDATION NOT ENOUGH

The standard recommendation of eight glasses (64 ounces) per day, in my opinion, is not nearly enough. You'll be surprised at how much more water you can—and should—drink.

Women in the Tighter Tummy groups in Gainesville drank 16 glasses (128 ounces) per day for the first week, and 20 glasses (160 ounces) per day for the second week. And you already know about their terrific fat loss results.

In addition to what it does to wash away fat from the waist, hips, and thighs, water is great for the skin. Many women have found that generous water consumption adds a smooth, supple, vibrant appearance to the complexion.

WATER YOUR FAT AWAY

Here is a list of exactly what to do to take advantage of the benefits of drinking more water.

- Purchase an insulated, 32-ounce, plastic container with a straw. Continuous sipping is more effective then gulping down a glass now and then. The straw enables you to consume more water than you can drink from a glass.

- Begin by consuming four 32-ounce containers a day for the first week. That's one gallon, or 128 ounces. Increase the amount to five containers, one-and-one-quarter gallons, a day for the second week.

- Keep track of your water drinking by placing rubber bands around the middle of the bottle equal to the number of containers of water you are supposed to consume. Remove a rubber band each time you finish 32 ounces.

- Try to drink 75 to 80 percent of the water before 5:00 p.m. That way you won't have to get up in the middle of the night to urinate. You will have to run back and forth to the bathroom very frequently during the day for the first week. However, during the second week, your bladder will become less sensitive and you will urinate less frequently but in larger amounts.

- Maximize calorie burn by keeping the water ice cold. A gallon of ice cold (40 degrees Fahrenheit) water requires over 200 calories of heat energy to warm it to core body temperature (98.6 degrees Fahrenheit). The insulated bottle will help keep the water chilled.

- Give your muscles a boost by drinking it while you exercise. From 70 to 75 percent of your muscle mass is composed of water. That's one reason you get thirsty when you exercise.

- Don't let your consumption of other liquids crowd out water. Regular coffee, tea, and soft drinks contain caffeine and other chemicals that may negate the benefits of water. You can actually decrease your taste for water by consuming too many flavored drinks.

- A sprig of mint or a slice of lemon or lime is all you need to spice up your water. Try it.

CRAVING WATER

"I've spent years feeling unsatisfied at the end of meals and trying to satiate my body with second helpings or desserts," said Kathryn Darden, who lost over ten pounds of fat on the Tighter Tummy Program.

"Now I realize what my body really needed was lots of water. Drinking water really satisfies my cravings."

Let's drink to it!

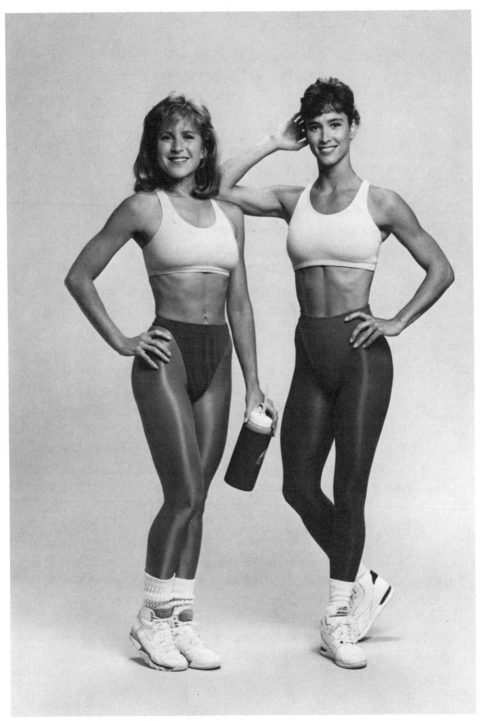

Muscle-building exercise is the most important component of the overall fitness practices of Jill Brooks and Jill McCann.

STEP 5

Emphasize Building Larger,
Stronger Muscles

M uscles are the least respected parts of the body. Even most physicians show little regard for them.

When the average woman has a thorough physical examination, her blood pressure and pulse rate are measured, her nervous system, eyes, and ears are examined, her blood and urine are analyzed, and her heart and lungs are examined. She is given an electrocardiogram, and x-rays are taken of whatever part of the body is suspected of being diseased or injured. This is as it should be.

But the patient's muscles are rarely examined. If tests *are* given, they gauge neurological deficiency. Tests to determine whether a woman's muscles can manage her body weight are uncommon, and so is an appraisal of flexibility and strength. Yet without muscles, the body cannot function.

MUSCLES PROVIDE CURVES

Without muscles your body would be a shapeless bag of bones with blobs of hanging fat surrounding your chest, belly, buttocks, and thighs. Muscles give interesting curves, sex appeal, and structural strength to your body.

Muscles also are directly related to your leanness and fatness. More than anything over which you have voluntary control, your muscles require calories—calories to keep warm, to contract, to stretch, to regulate, to recover, and to grow.

MUSCLES BURN EXTRA CALORIES

Add a pound of muscle to your body and you automatically require an extra 75 calories per day just to keep it alive. Add a pound of fat and your body needs only 2 calories a day to keep it functioning.

Muscle is 37.5 times more metabolically active than the same amount of fat. Lean women have a high muscle-to-fat ratio. Fat women have a low muscle-to-fat ratio. Their additional pounds of muscle are why lean women can consume so many dietary calories without getting fat compared with obese women who add fat on so few calories.

Thus, it makes sense to emphasize the building of larger, stronger muscles as you are losing fat. Fortunately, the best exercises for building your muscles also are the best ones for losing fat.

MUSCLE-BUILDING EXERCISE

There are a number of important principles you must understand and apply to make the recommended exercise as productive as possible.

Intense: Any exercise, to be meaningful, must be hard and demanding. Easy exercise does not fit the bill, no matter how long it is continued. Proper exercise must produce momentary muscular failure—until you cannot continue with the movement—within a time period of 60 to 180 seconds.

Progressive: There must be a practical way to make the exercise harder. In a two-week program you can do so by increasing the repetitions or the elapsed time. If you can perform an exercise continuously for 180 seconds, then you must add more resistance to the moving body part.

MISSI PIERCE

Age: 21

Height: 5'10"

Starting body weight: 144.8

Fat lost in pounds: 9.57

Inches lost from waist: 2³/₈

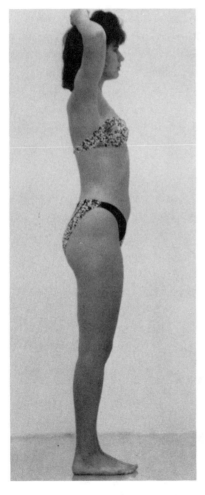

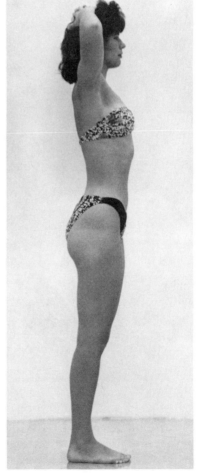

Before   *After*

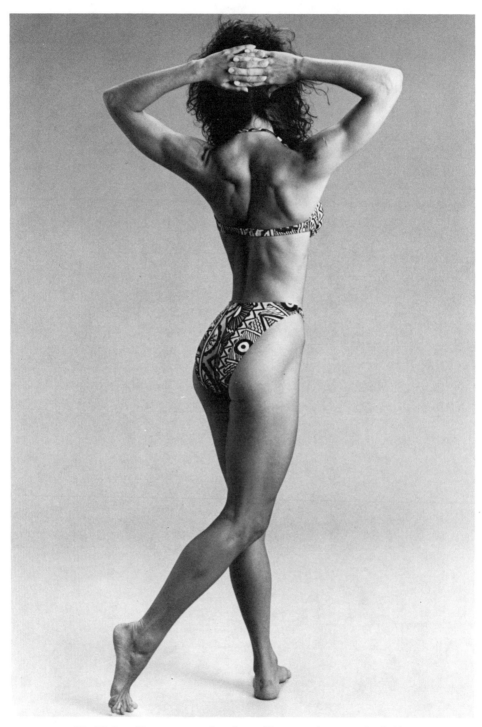

The Tighter Tummy exercise plan will **not** *neglect your backside.*

Form: Each repetition of every exercise should be performed slowly and smoothly. This will maximize the demands on the muscles and limit the role of momentum. While generating momentum is valuable in many athletic skills, it is counterproductive and dangerous in strengthening exercises. No quick and sudden movement is permitted. Special emphasis should also be placed on pausing and squeezing at the muscle's fully contracted position.

Frequency: The Tighter Tummy Exercise Routine is only practiced three times per week: Monday, Wednesday, Friday or Tuesday, Thursday, Saturday. Your body needs at least 48 hours of rest between major high-intensity workouts.

NO SPECIAL EQUIPMENT

It is easily possible to perform muscle-building exercise in the privacy of your home with no special equipment. If you can team up with a friend or several friends, your workouts will be even more effective. Some fitness centers in Florida, including the Gainesville Health & Fitness Center, offer Two Weeks to a Tighter Tummy under supervised conditions.

Regardless of the setting, your results should be similar to those of the women described in this book.

"Before the Tighter Tummy Program," says Jill Brooks, who registered a fat loss of 6 pounds, "I exercised too much. If I didn't do something every day I felt I would surely gain weight. But I learned the opposite is true. By giving my body a few days off each week to rest, I've increased energy and my overall figure and fitness are better than I can ever remember."

Get ready to strengthen your muscles and tighten your tummy.

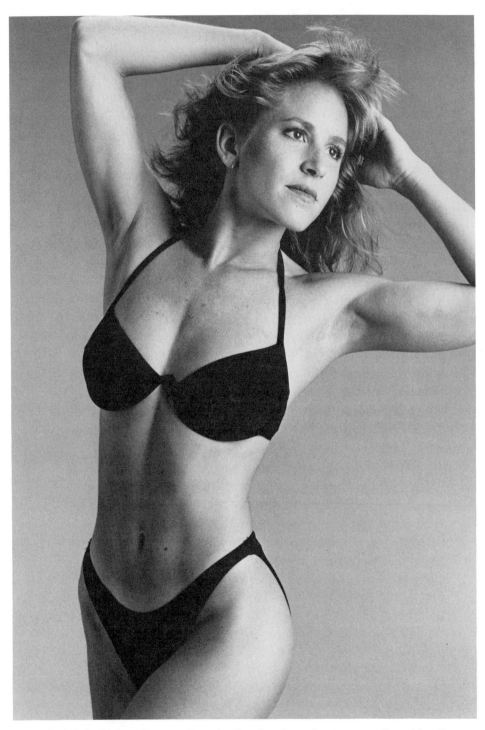

You'll feel the Tighter Tummy Exercise Routine throughout your entire midsection.

STEP 6

Isolate Your Abdominals with Proper Exercise

Many women believe that when you exercise a specific body part, such as the abdominals, the involved muscles use the surrounding fat for energy. This belief is the reason high-repetition sit-ups and leg raises have been practiced for years as a way to remove fat from the waist.

SPOT REDUCTION IS NOT POSSIBLE

If spot reduction of fat was possible, then people who chew gum regularly would have skinny faces. But such is not the case.

No direct pathways exist from the muscle cells to the fat cells. When fat is used for energy, it is mobilized primarily through the liver from multiple fat cells all over the body.

SPOT PRODUCTION OF STRENGTH

While spot reduction of fat from your waist is not possible, spot production of tightness and firmness is possible and highly recommended. Your goal is to make your abdominal muscles—*rectus abdominis, external oblique, internal oblique,* and *transverse abdominis*—significantly stronger, which in turn will make your entire tummy area tighter and firmer.

MUSCLE ISOLATION

The exercise routine illustrated in this chapter isolates and intensely works your abdominals, but it does not neglect other major muscles. You'll also be exercising your hips, thighs, chest, arms, and neck. This not only facilitates fat loss, but helps to balance your figure.

Combine the exercise routine with the other steps in this course and you've done everything practical—just short of surgery—to maximize tummy tightening.

PRECISION BASICS

The hardest thing about exercise is getting started. To jump from no exercise to exercise demands a big effort. Here are some hints that will make that hurdle easier.

Read through first: Spend several minutes looking over the exercises in this chapter. Read the directions carefully to get an idea of the routine. Practice will perfect your movements, but for now, do them as best you can.

Control your movements: Rushing through each exercise diminishes effects and can result in injury. Do each repetition slowly, smoothly, and intensely. Each exercise, with one or two exceptions, should take approximately 4 seconds on the lifting and 4 seconds on the lowering. If in doubt about your speed of movement, always move slower rather than faster.

Emphasize breathing: Try not to hold your breath on any exercise. Keep your mouth open and breathe. When the movement gets difficult, purse your lips and blow—just like they teach in a Lamaze class.

Count the repetitions: Start with 6 repetitions on most

exercises, then at each workout, increase the repetitions by 2. Thus, if you start your workouts on a Monday, the progression would be as follows:

Week 1	Monday	—	6 repetitions
	Wednesday	—	8 repetitions
	Friday	—	10 repetitions
Week 2	Monday	—	12 repetitions
	Wednesday	—	14 repetitions
	Friday	—	16 repetitions

After you can do 16 repetitions, or approximately 180 seconds of any movement, you must progress to harder forms of exercise.

Focus your concentration: Proper exercise is both physical and mental. Direct your attention to the muscles you're working and your results will improve. If it's a trunk curl, for example, focus on the front abdominals. Try to see them contracting in your mind each time you lift and lower. If it's a side bend, focus on mobilizing your oblique muscles to their maximum. Aim your mind like a laser beam. The effect will amaze you.

Expect some soreness: Soreness in exercised body parts is an indication that you've stretched and contracted some underutilized muscles. Expect some tenderness after your first workout, especially on your sides and abdomen. Don't fret. Your second workout will ease the soreness and it should be gone by your third exercise session.

TIGHTER TUMMY EXERCISE ROUTINE

The following routines can be performed with rhythmic music in the background. Do one set of nine exercises for the first week and one set of ten exercises for the second week. Neither of the routines should take longer than 30 minutes.

WEEK 1

1. Marching in place
   (warmup)
2. Side bend
3. Trunk curl
4. Trunk curl with twist
5. Hip flexion
6. Reverse trunk curl
7. Wide squat against wall
8. Negative pushup
9. Hip raise

WEEK 2

1. Marching in place
   (warmup)
2. Side bend
3. Trunk curl
4. Trunk curl with twist
5. Hip flexion
6. Reverse trunk curl
7. Wide squat against wall
8. Negative pushup
9. Hip raise
10. Reverse trunk curl

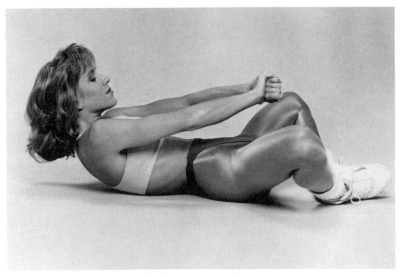

Trunk curl, contracted position.

TRUNK CURL

Day by day you'll see
those belly rolls flatten.
Give this exercise your best effort.

Starting position: Lie face up on floor. Bring heels close to buttocks and spread knees. Clasp hands over navel.

Movement: Curl shoulders gradually off floor and reach with hands between thighs. Only one-third of a standard situp can be performed. Pause briefly in top position. Lower shoulders slowly to floor. Repeat for required repetitions.

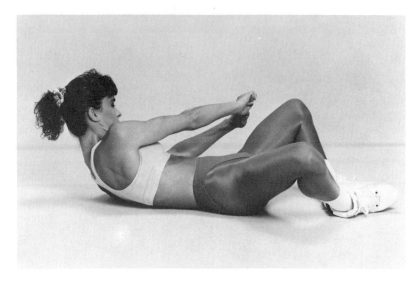

Trunk curl with twist, contracted position left.

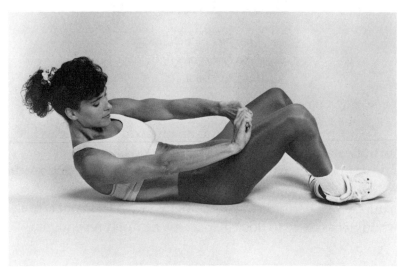

Trunk curl with twist, contracted position right.

TRUNK CURL WITH TWIST

*This curl-twist combo attacks
tummy flab like crazy—
and it makes your middle firm.
Don't hold back!*

Starting position: Assume same position as for trunk curl.

Movement: Curl shoulders gradually off floor and reach with hands toward left knee. In top position, twist slowly with torso to right and try to touch right knee. Lower shoulders smoothly to floor. Repeat movement, but this time reach to right knee, then twist to left, and lower. Alternate left-to-right and right-to-left twisting for required repetitions.

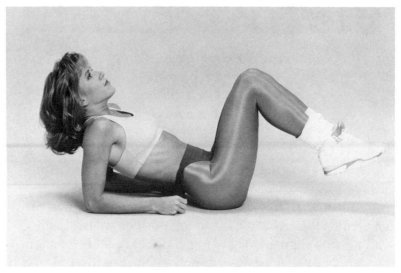

Hip flexion, midrange position.

HIP FLEXION

*There's nothing like the knee-up
to tone the tie-in area
between your hips and thighs.
Keep your lower back rounded.*

Starting position: Sit on floor. Lean back and support upper body on elbows. Straighten legs in front and keep feet and knees together.

Movement: Pull thighs slowly to chest by flexing hips and knees. Return thighs to extended position. Keep feet approximately six inches off floor during movement. Repeat for required repetitions.

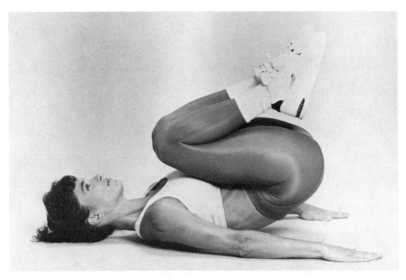

Reverse trunk curl, contracted position.

REVERSE TRUNK CURL

*That puffy pooch below your
navel can hang on stubbornly.
Here's a terrific exercise to help
dislodge it for good.*

Starting position: Lie face up on floor with hands, palms down, on either side of hips. Bring thighs on chest so hips and knees are in flexed position.

Movement: Curl pelvic area toward chest by lifting buttocks and lower back. Push down on floor with hands. Hips and lower back should be at 45 degree angle to floor. Lower hips smoothly to floor. Try not to cheat by moving feet or knees. Repeat for required repetitions.

After the reverse trunk curl, release tension in your abdominals by easing into a flowing stretch. Lie on your back with legs relaxed and arms over head. Take a deep breath, arch lower back, and expand rib cage. Exhale slowly and repeat several times.

Note: You'll do a second set of the reverse trunk curl at the end of each workout during Week 2.

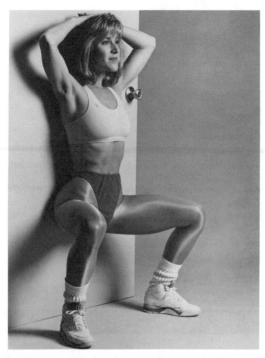

Wide squat against wall, bottom position.

WIDE SQUAT AGAINST WALL

*Cottage-cheeselike fat on your
hips and thighs is smoothed away
by this one nifty exercise.
Work through the burn and reap the results!*

Starting position: Stand erect and lean back against a smooth, sturdy wall. Place heels six inches wider apart than hips and approximately 12 inches away from wall. Adjust hands on top of head.

Movement: Bend at hips and knees and slide down wall until tops of thighs are parallel to floor. Hold for 10 seconds. Push back to top and immediately lower to parallel position. Do not lock knees in top position. Keep them bent slightly. Repeat for 5 sustained contraction repetitions. Increase the duration of each repetition by 5 seconds each workout. Your goal is to do five 30-second repetitions.

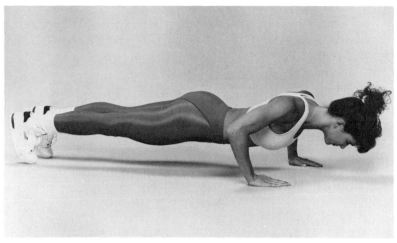

Negative pushup, midrange position.

NEGATIVE PUSHUP

*This improved version of the
classic pushup will firm and strengthen
your chest, shoulders, and arms.*

Starting position: This is the only exercise you'll do in a negative, or lowering-only, manner. Assume a standard pushup position on toes and hands with body stiff.

Movement: Lower body to floor by bending arms slowly in approximately 6 seconds. Do not try to push yourself up to top position. When you reach floor, bend knees, round back, straighten arms, get back on toes, and stiffen body once again. Repeat in the standard fashion for 6 repetitions. Add 2 repetitions per workout. Your goal in two weeks is to do 16 negative-only repetitions.

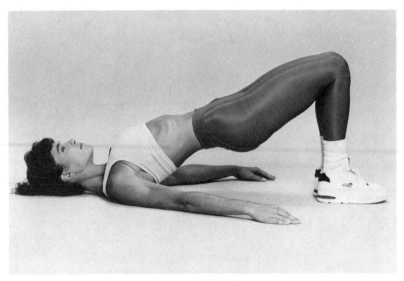

Hip raise, contracted position.

HIP RAISE

This exercise zeros in on tightening your tush. It's a winner in every woman's routine.

Starting position: Lie face up on floor. Slide feet under knees. Place hands, palms down, on either side of hips.

Movement: Raise hips upward. Keep head, shoulders, and hands on floor. Arch lower back slightly. Contract buttocks intensely. Lower hips back to floor. Repeat for required repetitions.

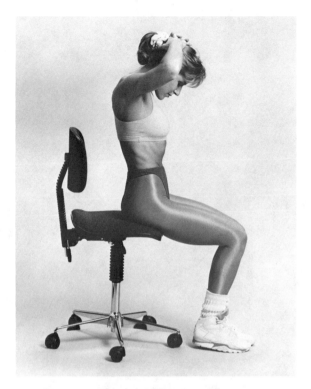

Neck extension, stretched position.

NECK EXTENSION

*A strong neck helps you carry
your head taller, creating a
longer silhouette.*

Starting position: This posture-pleasing exercise is performed at home on your non-exercise days, first thing in the morning and last thing before going to bed. Stand, interlace your fingers, and place hands on back of head.

Movement: Pull head forward with arm muscles while resisting the pull with neck muscles. When chin is on chest, reverse directions. Extend head backward and resist movement with hands and arms. Try to establish a fluid, smooth, continuous motion. Do 6 repetitions twice a day on each of your non-exercise days.

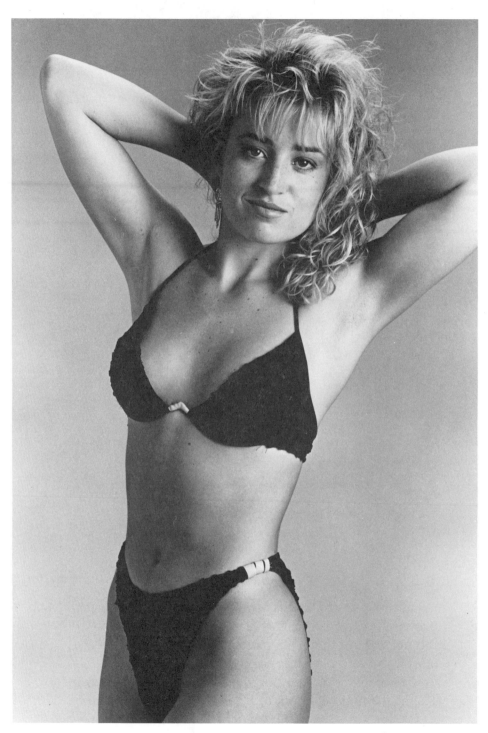

Laura Kelly added over three pounds of muscle to her shapely figure.

NON-EXERCISE DAYS

Let's say you're going to perform the Tighter Tummy Exercise Routine on a Monday-Wednesday-Friday schedule. You'll want to make certain that you get adequate rest on your non-exercise days—Tuesday, Thursday, Saturday, and Sunday—which will be fully described in Step 9.

While you'll do no serious, progressive, high-intensity exercise on these in-between days, I do recommend that you perform three exercises at home on these days. The exercises, all previously illustrated, are the:

- Side bend
- Trunk curl
- Neck extension

Perform them for one set of 6 repetitions, in the morning before breakfast and at night before bed. Do not progress in any of them. Always keep the repetitions at 6.

Such exercises will not make you significantly stronger. They will, however, contribute to making you aware of keeping your stomach tight, improving your posture, and standing tall.

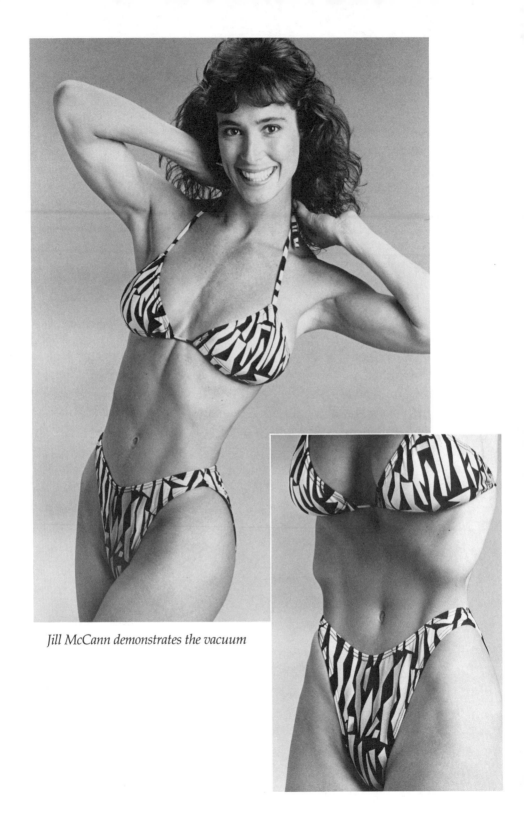

Jill McCann demonstrates the vacuum

STEP 7

Practice Doing a Stomach Vacuum

What is a stomach vacuum?

It is not a pump attached to a hose that goes down your throat to suck food out of your stomach. It is, however, a unique breath-holding feat that can help you to:

- Work your abdominals from the inside out
- Curb your appetite
- Flatten your stomach

The stomach vacuum is a trick I learned twenty years ago from a champion bodybuilder. When he was going through his on-stage posing routine, this bodybuilder could suddenly suck in his stomach and expand his chest to such a degree that you could almost see his backbone from the front. Then he could deflate his chest and pop out his clearly defined abdominal muscles one at a time from top to bottom.

It was an impressive display of muscle control and contributed greatly to this man's winning many physique contests.

While entering a bodybuilding contest is probably of no interest to you, learning to do the first part of a stomach vacuum is an important step in gaining control of your tummy.

KATHRYN DARDEN

Age: 21

Height: 5'7"

Starting body weight: 140

Fat lost in pounds: 10.36

Inches lost from waist: 3^1/$_2$

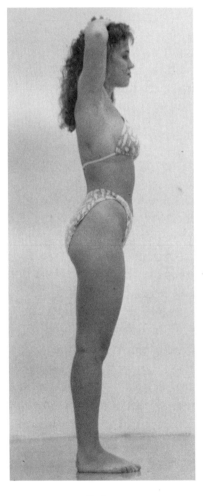
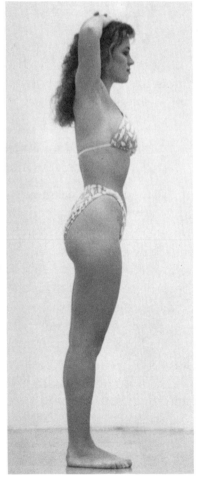

Before   *After*

STOMACH VACUUM SPECIFICS

To do a vacuum, you must have an empty stomach. It should be two hours or more since you've eaten. Here's what to do:

- Lie comfortably in bed on your back.
- Place your hands across the bottom of your rib cage and top of your abdominals.
- Take a normal breath and forcibly blow as much air out of your lungs as possible. This should take about 10 seconds.
- Suck in your stomach or belly to the maximum degree. It is important that you take no air in at this point. You should feel a concave formation under your rib cage. You won't be able to hold this vacuum feat very long. Three or four seconds is tops, at most.
- Practice the vacuum several more times while lying down. If you feel a little light-headed, that's normal. Rest a bit longer between trials.
- Stand now and get in front of a mirror and try the vacuum. Take off your shirt so you can see what's happening. At first, the vacuum is a little more difficult to do standing than lying, but with a little more practice, you should be able to master it in a standing position.

WHEN TO USE THE VACUUM

Practice the stomach vacuum twice before each major meal: breakfast, lunch, and dinner. In other words, you'll be doing it six times a day every day for two weeks.

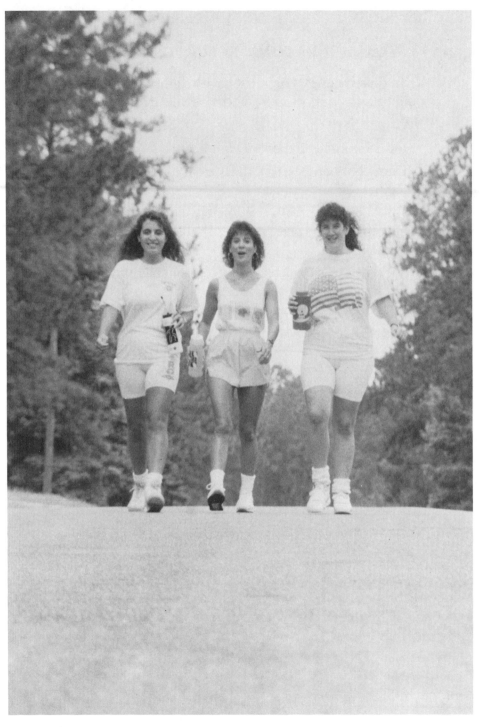

Walking after the evening meal speeds up the fat-loss process. During the two-week plan, Liz Guinta lost 8.45 pounds, Rosemarie Weaver lost 5.81 pounds, and Criss Cirulli lost 9.2 pounds of fat.

STEP 8

Walk After Your Evening Meal

I've never been much of a believer in walking as an effective method of exercise.

Walking does nothing for your strength or flexibility. It can produce a benefit on your cardiovascular endurance, but only if you walk uphill or at a fast speed. Even then, there are certain uphill-downhill dangers and impact forces that may offset the benefit.

Nor is walking an efficient way to burn calories. At least I didn't believe it was until I applied the results of a study by Dr. J. Mark Davis and colleagues from the Department of Exercise Sciences, University of South Carolina.

Dr. Davis measured and compared the energy expenditure for three hours of seven women after the following treatments: exercise only, meal only, exercise-meal, and meal-exercise. The results showed that the meal-exercise routine increased energy expenditure among the women by an average of 30 percent, compared with the other treatments. The researchers concluded that going for a walk after you eat brings on "exercise-induced post-prandial thermogenesis," which means the production of extra body heat created by exercising on a full stomach.

THERMOGENESIS—
THE PRODUCTION OF HEAT
The study by Dr. Davis's group got me thinking about

THERESA PEREZ

Age: 37

Height: 5'3"

Starting body weight: 118.5

Fat lost in pounds: 7.26

Inches lost from waist: 1$\frac{1}{2}$

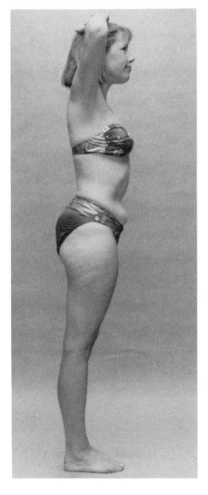

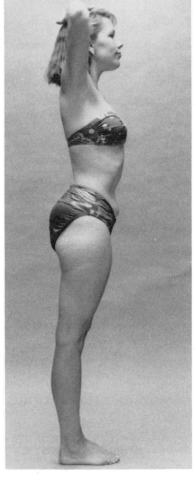

Before   *After*

thermogenesis. I decided to review the scientific literature on the subject. To my surprise, several other researchers had studied the effect and found that taking a walk after a meal can speed up heat production by as much as 50 percent.

Had anyone studied the thermogenic effect of eating, exercising, and drinking ice cold water as a subject walked? I could locate no references. But the more I thought about it, I realized that combining all three had to be an even better way of producing more heat and burning more calories.

THERMO-WALKING ROUTINE

After working with four groups of women at the Gainesville Health & Fitness Center, here's the thermo-walking routine that proved most effective:

- Eat your evening meal and drink your noncaloric beverage exactly as indicated in Step 2.
- Begin your walk within 15 minutes after you finish your meal.
- Walk at a leisurely pace for 30 minutes. How far should you walk at such a pace? A leisurely pace would cover from $1^1/2$ to 2 miles.
- Carry your insulated water bottle with you. Consume at least 16 ounces of cold water during the walk.
- Wear well-constructed, well-cushioned, and comfortable walking or running shoes. Do not wear street shoes. If you are unsure about which shoes to wear, go to your local athletic store and talk with a salesperson in the shoe department.
- Dress in lightweight, comfortable clothes when you walk.
- Walk outdoors, if possible, on level ground. Or you may substitute a bicycle ride for the walk. If the weather is a problem, you may walk indoors, or use an exercycle or treadmill.

MELTING FAT AWAY

Try the eating-walking-watering routine each day for two weeks and you'll be hooked on thermogenesis.

In a real sense you'll be melting fat away!

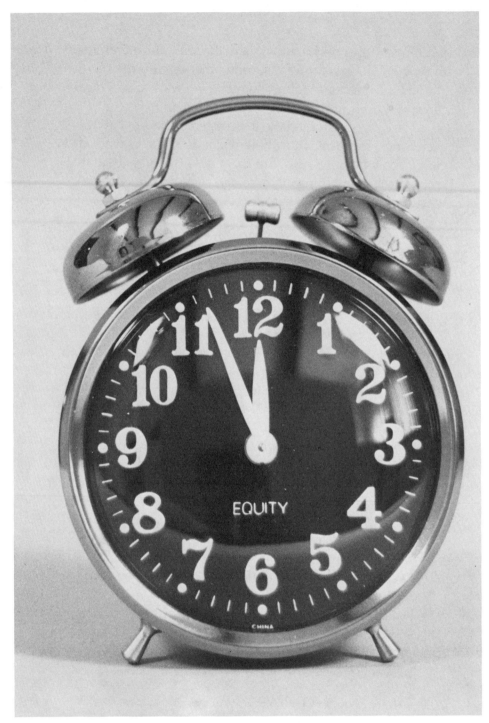

If you normally go to sleep at midnight, try to go to bed an hour earlier each night.

Step 9

Rest Adequately Each Day

Most days, do you feel tired or pooped?

If so, you're in the same bed with more than one-third of American adults. A recent Gallup Poll reported that one in three people are not getting enough sleep.

A similar survey conducted by *Glamour* magazine, but with the respondents being females between 18 to 35 years of age, found that 80 percent of these young women said they could use an extra hour or two of sleep each night. The main reasons for their lack of sleep were either work or school, followed by household tasks, social life, and children.

There's a good probability that you may fall into this category, that you could use more sleep each night. Sleep is especially essential if you're dieting and exercising. Efficient fat loss and efficient muscle building both require a well-rested recovery ability.

UNDERSTANDING RECOVERY ABILITY

Recovery ability is defined as the chemical reactions that are necessary for your body to produce efficient fat loss and muscle building. An optimum recovery ability is dependent on adequate rest, balanced nutrition, and sufficient time.

Your body is a complex factory, constantly making hundreds of delicate changes that transform food and oxygen into many chemicals needed by various parts of the system. But there is a limit to the chemical conversions that your recovery ability can make within a given time. If your requirements exceed that limit, your body will eventually be overworked to the point of collapse.

Thus, for maximum possible fat loss and muscle building, you must have the right combination of food, exercise, and rest. The combination doesn't work if you get too much or too little of any of the components.

SLEEP-REST FORMULA

Here's the formula concerning sleep and rest that worked so well with the women in Gainesville involved in the two-week plan:

- Go to bed an hour earlier each night, but get up at the same time as always each morning.
- Make sure your bedroom is dark, quiet, and comfortably cool.
- Place your alarm clock so you can't hear it ticking in the middle of the night.
- Don't eat or drink anything with caffeine in it after lunch.
- Avoid alcohol. It's not on the diet! Although alcohol is initially calming, it interferes with the soundness of sleep.
- Take a 15-minute nap during the middle of the afternoon, if possible.
- Shun vigorous activity on your non-exercise days. Do not participate in tennis, racquetball, running, aerobic dancing, Nautilus, or similar type of sports or fitness endeavors for the duration of this program.

REST NOW!

Apply the guidelines in this chapter, and not only will you improve your sleeping and resting, but you'll also facilitate your fat loss and muscle building.

Your dreams will soon be realities.

NOELLE GEIGER

Age: 34

Height: 5'4½"

Starting body weight: 114.7

Fat lost in pounds: 6.2

Inches lost from waist: 2¼

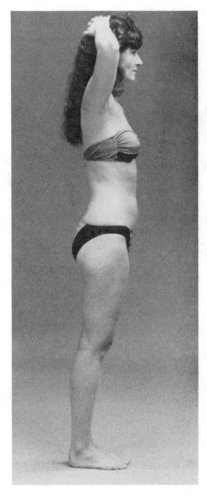

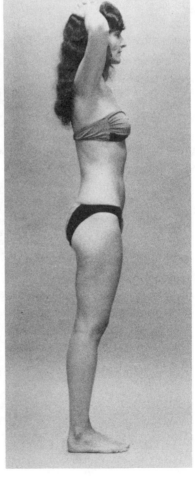

Before   *After*

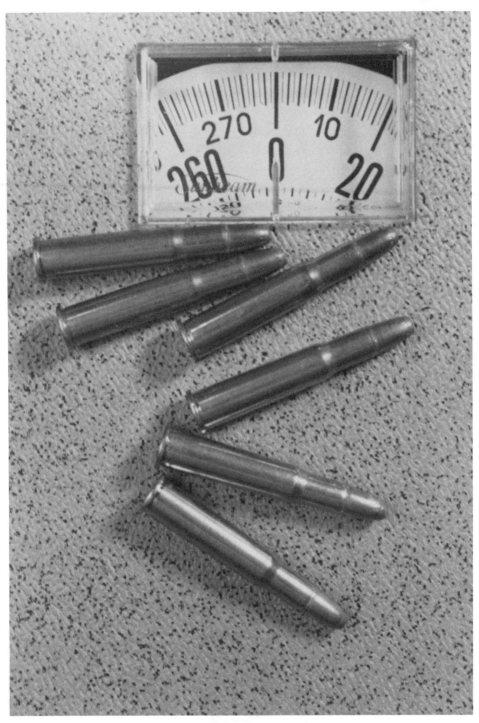

Let scientific ammunition help to conquer your weight-loss difficulties.

STEP 10

Combat Fat-Loss Problems with Facts

I n addition to Steps 1 through 9, there are a number of other facts that can help with the fat-loss process.

JOIN A SUPPORT GROUP

As previuosly mentioned, finding someone to go through the Tighter Tummy Program with you will be a big help. So will joining a support group. Two of the best support groups are Overeaters Anonymous and Take Off Pounds Sensibly (TOPS). Their local phone numbers should be listed in your phone book.

SLEEP COOL

Your body will burn significantly more calories each night if you sleep slightly cool. I'm convinced most people bury themselves under too many covers when they sleep. This prevents their normal thermostat from kicking in and supplying natural body heat.

If you tend to sleep with too many covers, try to eliminate one or two. Try to wean yourself from using an electric blanket and flannel sheets during the winter months, and

during the summer, try only a single sheet on top of you.
Soon you'll be burning several hundred more calories each
night and forcing your thermostat to work harder.

AVOID SAUNA, STEAM, AND WHIRLPOOL BATHS

Sauna, steam, and whirlpool baths heat the skin and
cause profuse sweating, which can lead to dehydration. Dehydration does not contribute to fat loss or fitness. In fact,
dehydration can actually cause your body to preserve fat.

Throughout this book, I've promoted keeping your
body well-hydrated and cool. Now, I'm advising you to stay
clear of products that cause excessive sweating.

PRACTICE GOOD POSTURE

Forget the traditional *stomach in, shoulders back* admoni-
tion. Even the U.S. Military Academy at West Point aban-
doned this so-called brace position in 1968 after an Army
study revealed it can cause a variety of problems.

The best posture resembles a marionette with a string
attached to the top of the head. Imagine being tugged gently
upward by the string. In other words, try to keep the top of
your head on the ceiling. Automatically this straightens out
the spine and tightens the abdominal muscles.

Practice sitting tall, standing tall, and walking tall.

BRUSH YOUR TEETH OFTEN

The next time you're really hungry, try brushing your
teeth. It's much harder to eat with a clean, minty taste in your
mouth. This is especially true if you crave something sweet
and you brush with a tingly toothpaste such as Ultra Brite.
The tingly taste will cause anything sweet to taste bitter tem-
porarily.

USE COLOR WISELY

Intense colors can stimulate your appetite. Don't use place settings or tablecloths of warm red, bright yellow, lime green, or orange. Even worse may be the red-and-white checkered tablecloths you often see in pizza parlors. You'll eat less on white or pastel plates and tablecloths.

CUT BACK ON YOUR EVENING TV

Watching television can hypnotize you to the point where you snack and don't realize how much you've eaten. Make it a personal rule never to eat while watching TV. Drinking water, getting outside for a walk, and going to bed an hour earlier will help you break the evening TV habit.

BEGIN A HOUSEHOLD PROJECT

To take your mind off food and keep your fingers busy, start a major project around the house. How about wall-papering the kitchen, refinishing a table, or needlepointing a pillow? Any number of other undertakings would be just as good. Get involved and your tummy tightening progress will soar.

VISUALIZE YOUR FUTURE FIGURE

Close your eyes and visualize the body you'd like to have. Allow your imagination a free reign. Practice this mind exercise twice a day as a motivating reminder of why you are struggling to change your eating and exercising.

BRIGHTEN YOUR BATH

Treat yourself to bath goodies like scented soap, aromatic shampoo, bubble bath, silky body lotion, and dusting pow-

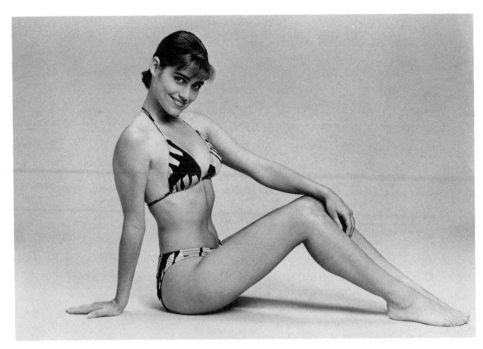

You'll be sitting pretty by the end of the two-week program.

der. These foster a sense of warmth and raise your body consciousness.

KEEP THE SCALE IN PROPER PERSPECTIVE

The scale can be a friend or foe. Obsession with the numbers can be self-defeating, since progress is often slow. Of the four research groups who went through the Tighter Tummy Course in Gainesville, the one that lost the most fat was the group who did not weigh during the program. It's probably demanding too much to ask you not to weigh yourself for two weeks, but if you can, do it. Realistically, however, try to weigh yourself no more than once a week.

BE ASSERTIVE

A leaner and stronger body automatically makes you more assertive. Practice saying *No!* when people offer you certain foods. Practice saying *Yes!* to things that are beneficial to your health. Soon you'll be in control—in *complete* control of your life.

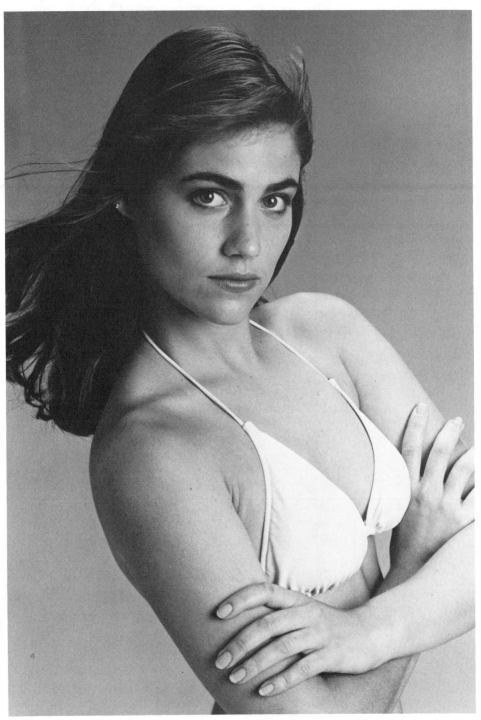

Specific instructions guided Kelli Jones towards her goals.

QUESTIONS AND ANSWERS

About Steps 1 Through 10

T he following questions were asked by women who went through the Tighter Tummy Program in Gainesville. The answers should clear up any areas of confusion you might have concerning the ten steps.

MEALS WITHOUT RED MEAT

Q. *I don't eat red meat. I notice that some of the Healthy Choice frozen dinners contain beef. What can I substitute for them?*

A. Three of the Healthy Choice dinners—Beef Pepper Steak, Salisbury Steak, and Lasagna—contain beef. The other four dinners—Chicken Enchilada, Breast of Turkey, Shrimp Creole, and Fettucini Alfredo—do not have beef in them. These four dinners should work well for two weeks.

If you still want more variety, try the Healthy Choice Macaroni and Cheese. It's in a 9-ounce frozen package and contains 280 calories. To complete the meal, add one slice of reduced-calorie bread (40), 2 teaspoons Heart Beat Spread (17), and $2/3$ cup of skim milk (60).

KELLI JONES

Age: 22

Height: 5'3$^{1}/_{2}$"

Starting body weight: 119.7

Fat lost in pounds: 8.4

Inches lost from waist: 2$^{1}/_{8}$

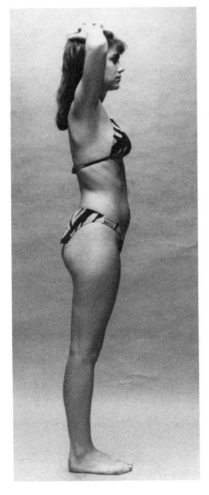
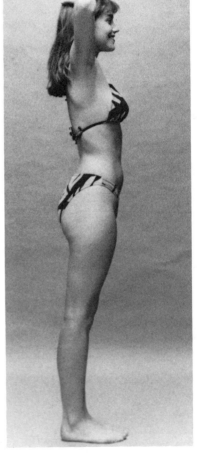

Before   *After*

ALLERGIC TO MILK

Q. *I'm allergic to milk. Can I still try your diet?*

A. Some health authorities estimate that as many as one in four adults have problems with the digestion of dairy foods. If you experience gas, bloating, or diarrhea after drinking milk, you may suffer from lactose intolerance. Typically, as many women enter their teens their bodies produce less lactose, the enzyme that aids in the digestion of the lactose in milk. This results in the distress you feel when you eat dairy foods.

Some of the research women who had this problem substituted light yogurt for skim milk. Others with the problem used a chewable tablet containing lactose that can be purchased at your supermarket.

DIET SALAD DRESSING

Q. *What kind of diet dressing do you recommend for the Chef Salad at lunch?*

A. There are many nonfat salad dressings available today at most supermarkets. What is called for on the Chef Salad at lunch is one which contains only 6 calories per tablespoon. A 6-calorie-per-tablespoon dressing is usually Italian. The Gainesville women mentioned most often that they liked Wishbone Lite Italian and Kraft Oil-Free Italian. Pritikin also makes a fat-free Italian dressing that is the only one I've seen that is sodium free.

SWITCHING DINNER AND LUNCH

Q. *Can I substitute dinner for lunch and lunch for dinner?*

A. Yes, as long as you don't make the switch more than once a week.

PUTTING WHOLE FAMILY ON PROGRAM

Q. *I'm a 40-year-old woman with a teenage son and daughter. My husband and I both want to lose 10 pounds and the children would also like to lose some weight. Can I put the whole family on your program?*

A. It would be great if you could, but you can't. The allowed calories per day is the problem. Men require significantly more calories each day than 1,100, and so do teenagers, who are still growing. Check with a registered dietitian (RD) for her recommendations. Steps 3 through 10, however, would apply to most men and teenagers.

USING CATSUP

Q. *Can I use catsup on your diet?*
A. No. Catsup contains calories and salt.

RAISINS EVERY DAY

Q. *I love raisins. Can I eat them every day for my snack?*
A. Yes, but I'd rather you vary the snacks. Many overweight women tend to be finicky eaters who dislike the taste of numerous vegetables and fruits. Try all the foods on this diet before you avoid certain ones. You just may discover that they have a place in your new eating lifestyle.

FOUR OR FIVE MEALS?

Q. *I weigh slightly more than 120 pounds. Would I be better off eating four meals a day, rather than the recommended five?*
A. No, stay with the five meals a day. Even if you weigh less than 120 pounds the day after you start the diet, stick with five meals.

HEADACHES

Q. *I often get headaches if I eat only 1,000 calories a day. What should I do?*

A. Your headaches may be caused by going longer than three hours between meals. Try saving some of your breakfast, lunch, or dinner for an in-between meal snack. For example, you could save a piece of reduced-calorie bread or a glass of skim milk for a later pick-me-up.

Some women who are used to drinking regular coffee notice headaches when they stop. If this applies to you, ease off the coffee more gradually.

Q. *I get a headache when I drink cold water. Can I drink water without it being chilled?*

A. Yes, but you won't get the 200-calories-or-more thermogenic effect from warming the cold water to core body temperature. Try a more gradual drinking of the cold water. You may have been consuming it too quickly.

DRINKING TOO MUCH WATER

Q. *Is it possible to drink too much water?*

A. Certainly, almost anything is possible, but to do so, you'd probably have to drink four or five times as much per day as I'm recommending. There are a few ailments, however, that can be negatively affected by large amounts of fluid. If you feel that you may have a problem, check with your personal physician before starting the program.

BOTTLED VERSUS TAP WATER

Q. *Is bottled water better than tap water?*

A. Research shows that bottled water is not always higher-quality water than tap water. The decision to drink bottled water or not is usually one of taste. If you dislike the taste of your tap water, then drink your favorite bottled water. If you have no problems with your city's water supply, then save money and consume it.

GRAMS OF FAT PER DAY

Q. *How many grams of fat should I eat each day?*

A. The Tighter Tummy Diet provides approximately 20 to 22 grams of fat per day. At 1,000 calories per day, approximately 18 to 20 percent of the calories are from fat. While you can certainly get too much fat each day from the food you eat, you can also get too little dietary fat. Twenty to 22 grams of fat per day works well for fat loss, nutritional well-being, and meal satisfaction.

TURNING FAT INTO MUSCLE

Q. *You talk about muscle and fat in Step 6. How does fat turn into muscle?*

A. Fat doesn't turn into muscle, and muscle doesn't turn into fat— not ever! The chemistry of each simply doesn't allow one to change to the other.

Both fat and muscle cells have the capacity to inflate or deflate. Like a balloon, they can swell or shrink. One of the goals of the Tighter Tummy Program is to decrease the size of your fat cells and increase the size of your muscle cells.

CHEWING GUM

Q. *Is it okay to chew gum during the two-week course?*

A. Yes, just make sure the gum does not contain sugar or calories. Do not, however, chew gum during your high-intensity exercise routines. It could disturb your focus of relaxing your face and breathing when the exercise gets hard.

Jennifer Griffin

Age: 29

Height: 5′3¹/₄″

Starting body weight: 132.3

Fat lost in pounds: 9.13

Inches lost from waist: 2¹/₂

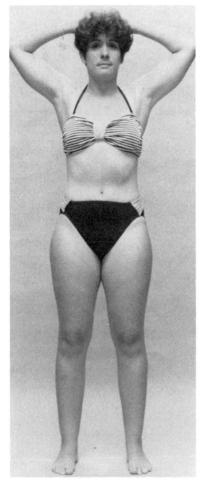
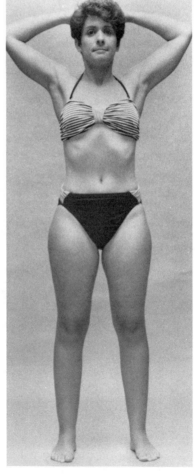

Before   *After*

RUNNING FOR WALKING

Q. *What about substituting running for the daily walk?*

A. No, running is too vigorous an activity. You also could easily upset your stomach if you tried to run immediately after your evening meal. The idea is to turn up your body heat without overstressing your digestion. Walking is the best choice.

EXTENDING THE WALK

Q. *Will I get better fat-loss results if I extend the walk past the recommended 30 minutes?*

A. Thirty minutes was chosen because it does not deplete significant amounts of your recovery ability. Remember, your body must be well rested to provide all the chemicals necessary for maximum fat loss and maximum muscle building to occur. It's easily possible on a low-calorie diet, if you're not careful, to start burning the candle at both ends. Do *not* walk more than the recommended 30 minutes.

FREQUENT BRUISING

Q. *I get black and blue marks on my legs when I diet. Am I doing something wrong?*

A. I doubt that you are doing anything wrong. Such black and blue marks are usually the result of an increased level of estrogen circulating in your body, which weakens the walls of the capillaries and causes them to break under the slightest pressure. When this happens, blood escapes and a bruise occurs. Estrogen is broken down in the liver, and so is fat. When you are dieting, your liver breaks down the fat, leaving a lot more estrogen in the bloodstream.

Supplementing your diet with 100 milligrams of vitamin C per day may help to toughen the walls of the capillaries.

AFTER MEASUREMENTS

Q. *When I finish the two-week program, should I retake my measurements?*

A. Absolutely! Turn back to page 18. Take the very same measurements, under the identical conditions, that you did two weeks earlier. Record the *After* measurements to the right of the *Before* measurements. Then subtract the *After* from the *Before* and record the number in the *Difference* column.

How did you do?
If you followed all the steps precisely, your results should be similar to the averages of the 100 women who completed the program at the Gainesville Health & Fitness Center.

Their averages were as follows:

Weight loss: -5.76 pounds
Muscle gain: +1.26 pounds
Fat loss: -7.02 pounds
Waist: (greatest of
     three positions):   -1.83 inches
Hips: -0.80 inches
Thighs: -1.37 inches
Total (six sites):   -6.08 inches

Anything close to these averages should have produced a significant tightening in your tummy. The next chapter shows you how to continue with the program.

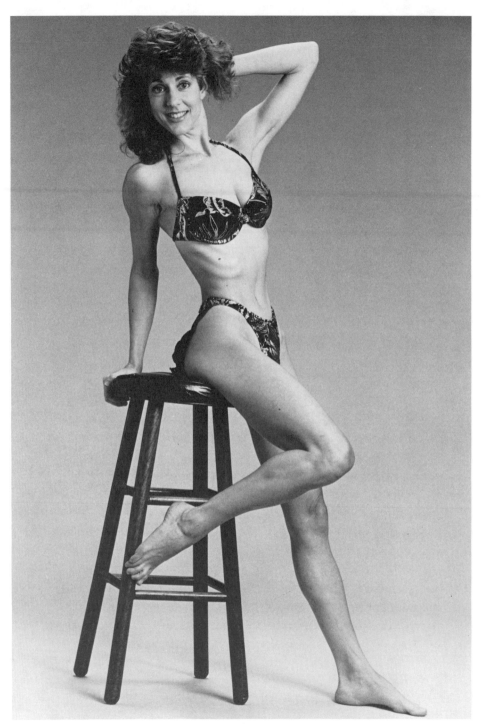

Of the 100 women who finished the two-week course in Gainesville, Cynthia Niemann had the smallest waist: $21^3/_8$ inches.

What to Do After Two Weeks

You're pleased with the results so far, but you still have a few more pounds and inches to lose. The most fat lost by any of the 100 women at the Gainesville Health & Fitness Center was 10.36 pounds.

If you had more than 10 pounds of fat to lose, you'll need to modify the ten-step program slightly to continue after two weeks. The primary steps that need modification are Step 2, the lower-calorie diet, and Step 6, proper exercise. All the other steps can be continued as you've practiced them for the last two weeks.

LOWER-CALORIE DIET

As I mentioned earlier, you should not consume 1,000 calories a day for longer than two weeks. If you do there's a high probability that your body will start using your muscle mass as a source of calories. When this happens, your body's calorie-burning potential will be lowered— and you'll become weaker and less energetic. It's simply not healthy.

What you must do is increase your daily calories by 200 (or 100 if you've been eating 1,100). Go up to 1,200 a day for the next two weeks.

WINSOME BENJAMIN

Age: 25

Height: 5'6¹/₂"

Starting body weight: 162.7

Fat lost in pounds: 10.34

Inches lost from waist: 3

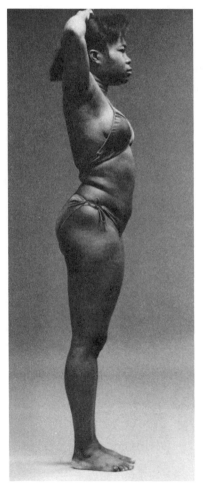
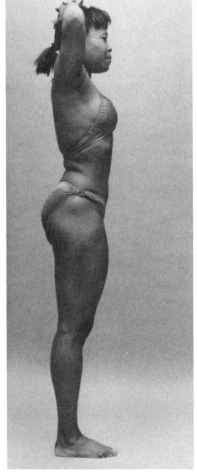

Before　　　　　　　　*After*

If you were pleased with the eating plan in this book, all you have to do is add 100 calories to the breakfast and another 100 calories to the lunch selections. A fruit serving of approximately 100 calories is the preferred addition.

Below are popular fruits, their serving sizes, and their calorie counts. You'll have to select your daily fruit choices to equal approximately 200 calories.

1 cup unsweetened applesauce (106)

1 cup apple juice (116)

1 cup canned apricots, juice pack (119)

10 dried apricot halves (83)

1 cup fruit cocktail, juice pack (115)

1 cup unsweetened grapefruit juice (96)

10 grapes, Thompson seedless (35)

$^1/_2$ cantaloupe (5-inch diameter) (94)

1 nectarine (2$^1/_2$-inch diameter) (67)

1 orange (2$^1/_2$-inch diameter) (55)

1 cup orange juice (111)

1 peach (2$^1/_2$-inch diameter) (37)

1 cup canned peaches, juice pack (109)

1 Bartlett pear (2$^1/_2$-inch diameter) (98)

1 cup canned pears, juice pack (123)

1 cup pineapple, juice pack chunks (150)

1 cup unsweetened pineapple juice (140)

1 plum (2$^1/_8$-inch diameter) (36)

1 cup canned plums, juice packed (146)

5 dried prunes (100)

1 cup prune juice (181)

1 cup strawberries (45)

1 tangerine (2 $^1/_2$-inch diameter) (45)

If you want to try another great eating plan that requires a bit more preparation time, get a copy of *Hot Hips & Fabulous Thighs*, also available from Taylor Publishing. It contains a terrific 1,200-calorie-a-day diet along with some great recipes.

After two weeks of 1,200 calories a day, descend the calories by 100 for another two weeks, and yet another 100 for a final two weeks.

In other words, the extended eating plan is as follows:

Weeks 1 & 2: 1,000/1,100 calories per day
Weeks 3 & 4: 1,200 calories per day
Weeks 5 & 6: 1,100 calories per day
Weeks 7 & 8: 1,000 calories per day

This plan should give you ample time to lose your excess pounds and inches. Then you'll be ready to progress to the maintenance program in the next chapter. In the meantime, I suggest that you read *Hot Hips & Fabulous Thighs* for more advice about my six-week, descending-calorie diet.

PROPER EXERCISE

The Tighter Tummy Exercise Routine described in Step 6 is only effective for a short time. Soon the involved muscles become strong enough to exceed the recommended repetitions or time span. Once you can perform more than 16 continuous repetitions, or more than 3 minutes of any exercise, you must progress to harder exercise. Your body weight alone does not supply enough resistance for your increasingly stronger muscles. I suggest that you progress to barbells, dumbbells, and weight machines.

Visit your local fitness center or YMCA/YWCA and ask them for help. They should be able to steer you in the right direction. Or you can read two of my previous books: *The Six-Week Fat-to-Muscle Makeover* and *The Nautilus Book*.

Many of the women who finished the research program at the Gainesville Health & Fitness Center have settled on an exercise routine that includes:

- Nautilus machines on Mondays and Fridays
- Floor exercises for the tummy and hips, similar to those in Step 6, on Wednesdays.

I suggest that you do the same until you reach your goal.

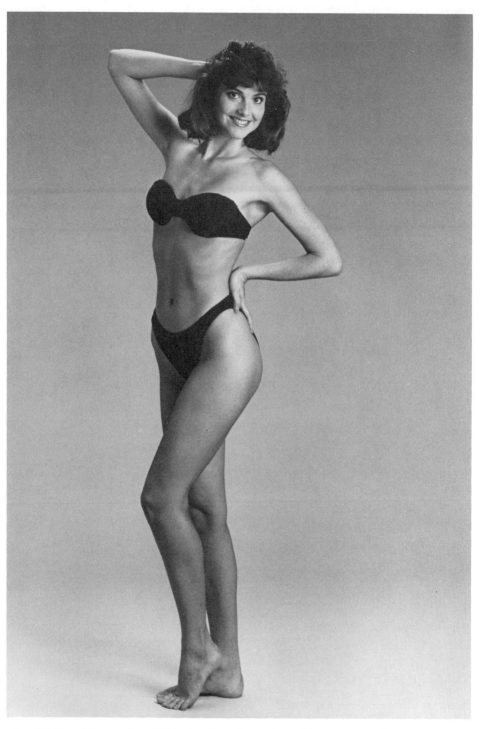

Cynthia Berg-Herman lost 2⁷/₈ inches from her waist and has kept it off by applying the mechanics in this chapter.

MAINTENANCE:
Keeping It Off

Now that you've tasted success, you don't want to give up your trim middle and sleek new body.

Rebound gaining, however, is all too common. Some experts note as many as 95 percent of all dieters fail to maintain their losses.

Dismiss these statistics. If you understand the steps—and make a continued effort—you'll never be bothered by belly fat again.

It's time to make the transition from losing to maintaining by returning to the ten steps.

STEP 1. EAT SMALLER MEALS MORE FREQUENTLY

You've been limiting your four or five meals per day to 400 calories or less per meal, to maintain your body weight, set the limit per meal at 500 calories or less. A 500-calorie meal will still keep your insulin responses small. Furthermore, 500-calorie meals are something you can easily adapt to—at least, most of the time.

What happens when you occasionally eat more than 500 calories at one time? Don't panic. Simply understand that you are human and that you will sometimes backslide. Learn to anticipate these urges and take corrective actions.

There is no disgrace in backsliding. The disgrace is in letting a lapse get you so discouraged that you quit trying. Don't let this happen to you.

Move forward immediately and get back on track with 500-calorie meals.

STEP 2. ADHERE TO A LOWER-CALORIE, CARBOHYDRATE-RICH DIET

Your lower-calorie diet can now be raised to the moderate-calorie level. Instead of consuming from 1,000 to 1,200 calories per day, you'll be eating from 1,500 to 2,200 calories per day. Maybe you can eat even more after your new body weight has stabilized.

There is no simple way to determine in advance how many calories you will need to maintain your new body weight. Trial-and-error experimentation will make the level obvious, however.

You should probably begin with 1,700 calories per day and see what happens after a week. If your body weight keeps going down, raise the calories to 1,800 or 1,900, depending on how much weight you lose during the last week. Soon, you should reach a level where your body weight stabilizes. That level is *your* daily calorie requirement.

Try to keep your calories rich in carbohydrates. The 60:20:20 ratio of carbohydrates, proteins, and fats is not only ideal for losing fat, but is also ideal for maintenance. Fruits, vegetables, breads, and cereals are your primary sources of carbohydrates. On your maintenance eating plan, strive each day to consume six servings of fruits and vegetables and six servings of breads and cereals. Doing so will usually allow your other foods—meats and dairy products—naturally to fall into correct ratio.

An occasional unbalanced ratio, or significant calories above your maintenance level, draws the same response discussed in Step 1. Accept the fact that you're human and these things will happen. Anticipate, plan, and get back on track.

JOY RICHMOND

Age: 39

Height: 5'5$\frac{1}{2}$"

Starting body weight: 123.3

Fat lost in pounds: 6.22

Inches lost from waist: 2$\frac{3}{8}$

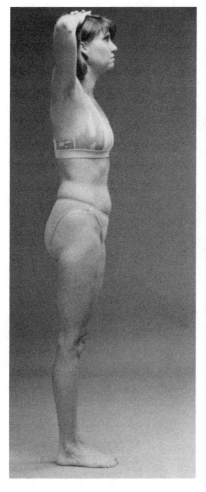

Before

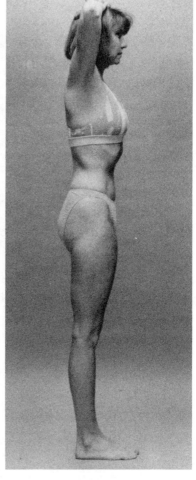

After

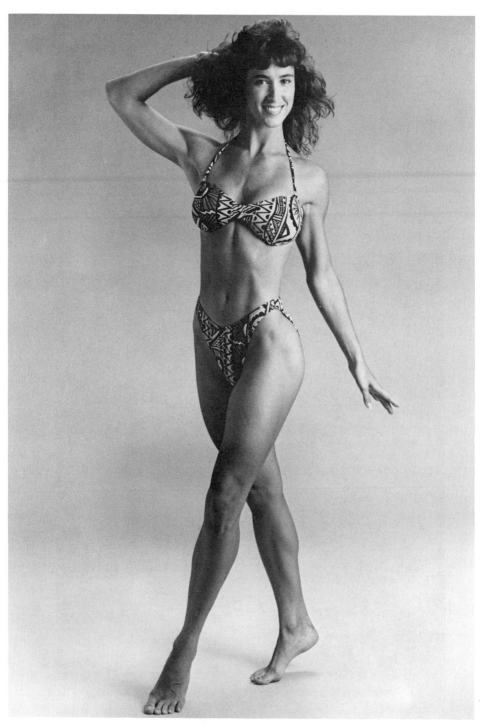

A great midsection contributes to a vibrant lifestyle.

STEP 3. REDUCE YOUR SALT (SODIUM) INTAKE

Keeping your sodium intake per day at 2,400 milligrams or less is an excellent guideline to follow on your maintenance plan. Become a conscientious reader of food labels. Take note of any serving of food that contains more than 600 milligrams of sodium. Be careful to avoid eating this food too often.

STEP 4. DRINK ONE TO ONE-AND-ONE-QUARTER GALLONS OF WATER PER DAY

I hope by now you've seen and felt the benefits of drinking plenty of ice cold water each day. Make it a permanent step in your new lifestyle to consume at least one gallon of water each day, and more when you can.

STEP 5. EMPHASIZE THE BUILDING OF LARGER, STRONGER MUSCLES

You never outgrow your need for larger, stronger muscles. Bigger muscles improve performance, add shape, stabilize joints, and burn more calories. Keep training them intensely and progressively and you'll be greatly rewarded.

STEP 6. ISOLATE YOUR ABDOMINALS WITH PROPER EXERCISE

Proper exercise to strengthen your abdominals—as well as other muscles— requires slow, focused movement. Slow, focused movement isolates your involved muscles, which in turn leads to firmness and tightness.

The primary difference between muscle-maintenance and muscle-building routines is that you do not need to work out as frequently in maintenance. To maintain muscle you only need to exercise two times per week. And you do not need to be progressive in adding resistance and repetitions.

A Nautilus machine workout or a barbell-dumbbell workout once or twice a week is recommended. Floor exercises for the abdominals once a week would be great, too. The early-morning and late-night movements at home on your non-exercise days are optional. You can always reinstate them, however, anytime your tummy starts getting a bit soft.

STEP 7. PRACTICE DOING A STOMACH VACUUM

This muscle-control feat can be used during maintenance to keep your appetite in the sensible range. Remember, twice before a major meal will put you in the driver's seat, rather than the other way around.

STEP 8. WALK AFTER YOUR EVENING MEAL

Walking on a full stomach is a great way to relax and burn significant calories. Don't forget to drink cold water while you walk to get the full thermogenic effect. You should take advantage of this effect often during your maintenance plan.

STEP 9. REST ADEQUATELY EACH DAY

Perhaps maintenance doesn't call for as much attention to rest as does losing fat. But since many women say they could use extra sleep, it certainly will be to your advantage to go to bed an hour earlier each night you can.

STEP 10. COMBAT FAT-LOSS PROBLEMS WITH FACTS

A dozen helpful facts were discussed is Step 10. Review them often and apply them anytime they are needed during your maintenance program. Your arsenal should now be well-stocked against any future fat-loss problems.

SYNERGY IN ACTION

- Synergy is defined as the simultaneous actions of separate parts, which together, have greater total effect than the sum of their individual effects.
- Synergy happens in your body when you combine Steps 1 through 10 into your day-to-day lifestyle.
- Synergy is why you now have a tight tummy.
- Synergy is why you'll have a tight tummy permanently.

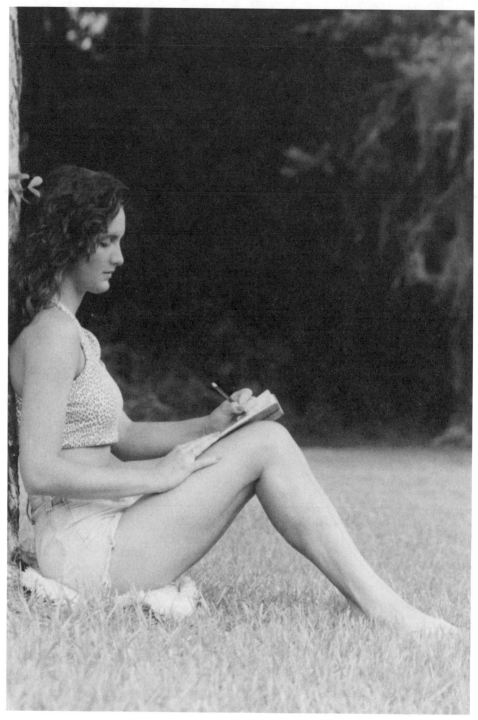

Organizing a daily diary allowed Katrine LaCroix to focus her attention on each of the ten steps.

A Personal
Diary

T he following is a day-by-day diary that Katrine
LaCroix kept as she went through the two-week program.
You'll probably find that many of her feelings are similar to
those that you experienced.

For the record, Katrine is a 21-year-old student at the
University of Florida. She began the program weighing 149
pounds and finished at 138.7, for a weight loss of 10.3
pounds. Katrine is one of seven women, out of 100, who lost
over 10 pounds. Here are her thoughts as she worked
through the course.

SUNDAY, JUNE 9

First official day of the Tighter Tummy Program. Bought the food yesterday after the body measurements and photos. Even got Ultra Brite, which leaves a tart taste for a while after brushing. Practiced the stomach vacuum and taught it to my mom. Drank a gallon of water and went to the restroom 20 times. Enjoyed my evening stroll. Went to bed feeling tired.

MONDAY, JUNE 10

Cold water seems to give me a mild headache. Ate a Dannon Light Yogurt for snack. My period began today but hardly any cramps—my insides are swimming in all the water. Great Chef Salad for lunch. Low energy level, especially after the exercise routine, which I felt. Took my 15-minute nap. Extra rest is needed! Felt better in the evening. Strange to try sleeping cool.

TUESDAY, JUNE 11

Felt at-home exercises for the first time. My own body weight feels tremendous. Still drinking the water, however. Forgot the milk that went with dinner. Had it after Ultra Brite: tasted repulsive. My period is almost over—very light. Nice to not have felt so cranky this month. Little energy at bedtime—sleepy early. Am I going to make it through this thing?

WEDNESDAY, JUNE 12

Another mild headache this morning. It went away after lunch. Exercise class was tough since I was sore, especially my midsection, from Monday's workout. Am getting a little used to all the water, a few less toilet trips. Ten-minute nap after exercise class picked me back up. I think the Fettucini Alfredo dinner's the best so far. Food sure tastes better when you're truly hungry.

KATRINE LACROIX

Age: 21

Height: 5′9¹/₂″

Starting body weight: 149

Fat lost in pounds: 10.3

Inches lost from waist: 2

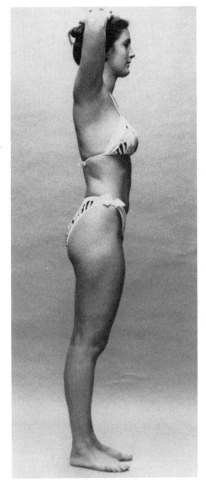

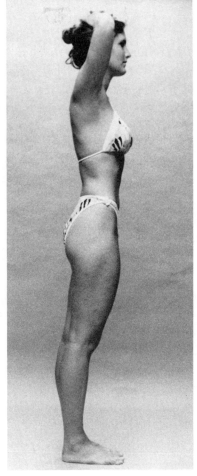

Before   *After*

THURSDAY, JUNE 13

Grandparents visited today. Mom got me to show them the vacuum trick. Mom even said she could see my cheekbones better. She and Grandma were commenting on my neck and collarbones being pretty—first time I'd heard that one. My rings have gotten looser. Had to switch them over to different fingers. Still feeling tired and not too energetic but sure feels good to be getting somewhere. I can really feel my waist shrinking.

FRIDAY, JUNE 14

Dr. Darden won't allow any of our group on a scale. I'm glad cause I think we're already too consumed with numbers. He says the weekend's the most difficult. If we can make it through to Monday, we're supposedly home free. I'm getting a few bruises on my thighs. Dr. Darden says it's normal if you're losing fat because of the increased estrogen level in the body. They come from fat being broken down in the liver, so I guess I don't mind the bruises too much. Exercise class went well. Our group seems determined to work hard. Wall squats are dreaded by everyone. My fingernails have gotten so strong and healthy looking. Wish I had the energy to paint them.

SATURDAY, JUNE 15

I've noticed my body temperature staying so much cooler from all the cold water—that's nice in the heat while everyone else is sweating. I like eating the smaller meals—keeps me feeling lighter. GOOD NEWS: I fit into some jeans I haven't worn in a year! Mom said my wrists even look smaller. Dr. Darden was right, the weekend is hard cause we're out of exercise routine. But I'm feeling more determined now, especially since my waist is shrinking a little each day.

SUNDAY, JUNE 16

Energy level actually rose today! Experienced no headaches and got a lot accomplished. Tried on a dress I haven't fit into in three years—not bad at all. Am beginning to see how imbalanced my meals were before this diet. I rarely took in enough fat. Didn't realize our bodies require it. Plus my meals were too large—I don't need that much.

MONDAY, JUNE 17

Body temperature still cool. Have almost constant goose bumps. Exercise class went well. I'm getting stronger. Enjoyed my evening walk. Seems much healthier to not eat late at night. I now even crave a lot of water if I don't have my bottle with me. Plus, I just know my weight is down—way down. Feels great to have beaten the weekend.

TUESDAY, JUNE 18

Big exam in school tomorrow. Studied a lot and ate dinner kind of late. It was too dark to walk—so I moved around inside my apartment trying to get that thermal effect Dr. Darden explained to us. I've cut out caffeine and have noticed fewer big ups and downs. Didn't sleep enough because of school—have to take a double nap tomorrow.

WEDNESDAY, JUNE 19

Made it through my exam. Relaxed out in the sun and my bathing suit fits so much better (not as tight). The water drinking has become almost a habit. Even kept me cool while sunbathing. Grandma said we'd have to go shopping once the program is over. I can really feel all the steps contributing now.

THURSDAY, JUNE 20

Still feeling terrific. Fingernails are pretty, as I finally painted them. Mom says my skin looks healthier. Been busy with school. The Lunch Bucket is handy when on the run and also tastes good. I've gotten attached to my morning "Go." Think I may keep those in stock too. Last exercise class tomorrow. I'm looking forward to it!

FRIDAY, JUNE 21

A very long day—three exams and the last exercise class. It was easier to work harder today, perhaps knowing it was the last session, or maybe my body's adjusting a bit. Anxious to get measurements tomorrow. Getting easier to fall asleep on an empty stomach. So glad to have taken part in this research. Learned a lot about water's importance and a well-balanced diet. Both are very necessary.

SATURDAY, JUNE 22

WOW! I did it. I not only survived the two weeks, but feel wonderful. Neat to see our group of women so pleased with the results. All seemed to carry themselves with a bit more pride and even stood taller. Enjoyed the smiling faces and was especially happy to have lost 10 pounds of body fat. And my waist is almost 24 inches. Hasn't been that small since tenth grade.

Grandma took me shopping this afternoon. Got the giggles in the fitting room cause she returned three times with a smaller pair of jeans. Finally bought a size 6—not a 9/10!! Hurray!

PREVENTING HEADACHES

I believe the mild headaches that Katrine noted during the first several days wouldn't have occurred if her total calories per day would have been 1,100 instead of 1,000. Her group of research subjects all consumed 1,000 calories per day. An additional 100 calories was not allowed for those women who started the program weighing over 120 pounds.

In other groups, when the extra 100-calorie snack was utilized, the participating women seldom noted a headache.

Too few calories can cause problems. Thanks, Katrine, for reinforcing this valuable lesson to me.

A special thank you also goes to Katrine for permitting me to share her personal diary with you. I hope the Tummy Tightening Program provides a lasting experience for her. And I hope you profit from her feelings and comments.

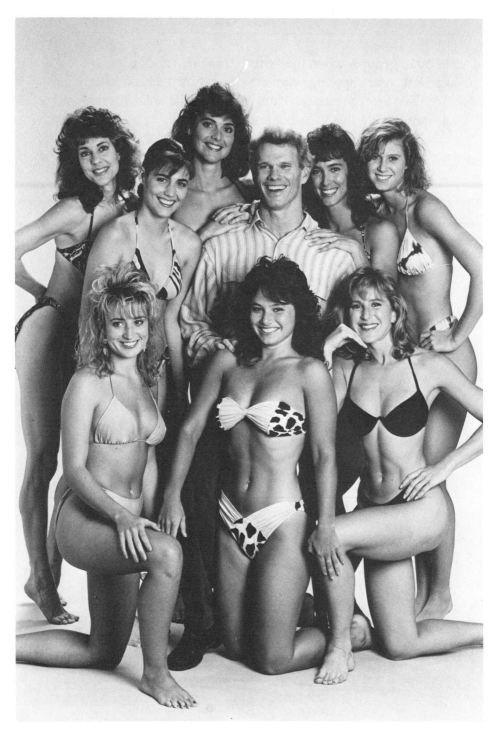

This picture was taken after a photo session in Orlando, Florida. Ellington Darden is in the middle with the forced smile.

PERMANENTLY TIGHT

T o keep your tummy permanently tight, you must have the discipline to apply Steps 1 through 10—not only for two weeks or two months—but for the rest of your life.

I want you to take to heart some advise borrowed from Zig Ziglar:

> "Life demands before it rewards. You've got to *be* before you can *do*, you've got to *do* before you can *have*. When you're tough on yourself, life becomes easy . . . You don't pay the price for good health, you enjoy the benefits of it—you pay the price for poor health."

You're enjoying the benefits of having a tight tummy.

Continue to be tough on yourself. With preparation and patience— you *can* do it.

Stay tight permanently!

ABOUT THE AUTHOR

Ellington Darden inspires many women with his disciplined approach to eating and exercising. His delivery is direct, his words are well-chosen, and his instruction is serious.

"After our first week of exercise classes," remembers one of the Tighter Tummy participants, "I thought he'd be perfectly cast as a Marshal in the old West. Even his sense of humor fits the impression: it's as dry as the plains.

"His stern, excuse-proof attitude, however, worked on me—as well as with the others in our group. I just wish he'd smile a little more."

Smiling more on the inside than on the outside, Dr. Darden focuses on his life's quest: to help people live leaner and stronger longer. He is the author of 36 books, which include *The Nautilus Diet, 32 Days to a 32-Inch Waist,* and *Hot Hips & Fabulous Thighs.* He also writes a popular column that appears in the Dallas Times Herald.

Recently, Dr. Darden's contributions were recognized when he was honored as one of the top ten health leaders in the United States by the President's Council on Physical Fitness and Sports.

Dr. Darden has been director of research for Nautilus Sports/Medical Industries since 1973. He holds bachelor's and master's degrees in physical education from Baylor University, and a doctor's degree in exercise science from Florida State University. Two years of post-doctoral study in food and nutrition set him on the trail that led to this book, which is the outgrowth of seven years of concentrated study.

Currently, Dr. Darden is doing research at the Gainesville Health & Fitness Center in Gainesville, Florida.